Michael Helfferich/Walther Hohenester

Homeopathy

Self-Healing Handbook

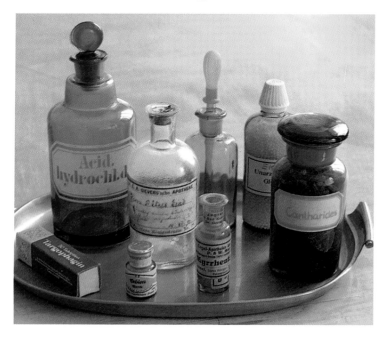

Sterling Publishing Co., Inc.

New York

Contents

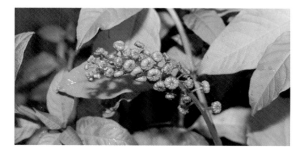

Phytolacca–*Pokeweed*

Library of Congress Cataloging-in-Publication Data

10 9 8 7 6 5 4 3 2 1

Published by Sterling Publishing Company, Inc.
387 Park Avenue South, New York, N.Y. 10016
Originally published and © 1997 by Südwest Verlag GmbH
& Co. KG, München under the title *Homöopathische
Hausapotheke*
English translation © 1999 by Sterling Publishing Co., Inc.
Distributed in Canada by Sterling Publishing
^c/o Canadian Manda Group, One Atlantic Avenue, Suite 105
Toronto, Ontario, Canada M6K 3E7
Distributed in Great Britain and Europe by Cassell PLC
Wellington House, 125 Strand, London WC2R 0BB, England
Distributed in Australia by Capricorn Link (Australia) Pty Ltd.
P.O. Box 6651, Baulkham Hills, Business Centre, NSW 2153,
Australia

Sterling ISBN 0-8069-5910-X

Foreword   4

**The Healing Principles
of Homeopathy**   6
Self-healing powers are activated   6
The potencies   8

**Symptoms and Ailments
    from A to Z**   12
Abdominal Pain   12
Abscess, Suppuration   13
Acne   15
Appetite Disorders   17
    - loss of appetite
    - excessive appetite
Backache   18
Bladder and Kidney
    Inflammation   20
Bad Breath   22
Burns   22
Canker Sores   25
Catarrh   26
Colds   28
Conjunctivitis   28
Constipation   31
Bronchitis Coughs   32
Chest Coughs   36
Diarrhea   38
Earache   41
Eczema   43
Fainting   44
Fever   45
Flatulence   47
Flu-like Symptoms   48
Gallbladder Problems   50
Bleeding Gums   51

Hangover, Overeating 52
Heartburn 52
Hemorrhoids 54
Hoarseness 55
Insect Bites and Stings 58
Insomnia 59
Lumbago 60
Nervous Disorders 61
Neuralgia 62
Overweight 63
Restlessness 65
Sciatica 66
Shoulder Pain 67
Sprains, Strains 68
Stomachache 69
Sunburn 71
Sunstroke 72
Tendinitis 74
Sore Throat 75
Travel Sickness 76
Voice Loss 78
Vomiting 79
Weather Sensitivity 80

The 31 Most Important Remedies 81

Aconitum napellus, Aconite
  (Monk's hood) 81
Allium cepa (Red onion) 81
Apis mellifica (Honeybee) 82
Arnica montana (Leopard's bane) 82
Arsenicum album (Arsenic
  trioxide, White arsenic) 83
Belladonna (Deadly nightshade) 83
Bryonia alba (Wild hops, White
  bryony) 84
Carbo vegetabilis
  (Vegetable charcoal) 84
Chamomilla (German chamomile)84
China (Peruvian bark) 85
Ferrum phosphoricum (Ferrum
  phosphate) 85
Gelsemium (Yellow jasmine) 85
Ignatia amara (St. Ignatius bean) 86
Kali bichromicum (Potassium
  bichromate) 86
Kali carbonicum (Potash,
  Potassium carbonate) 86
Lachesis (Bushmaster snake) 86
Ledum (Marsh tea) 87
Lycopodium (Club moss) 87
Magnesium phosphoricum
  (Magnesium phosphate) 88
Mercurius solubilis (Mercury) 88
Natrium muriaticum (Sodium
  chloride, table salt) 89
Nux vomica (Poison nut) 89
Phosphorus (Phosphorus) 90
Pulsatilla (Wind flower) 90
Rhus toxicodendron (Poison ivy) 91
Ruta graveolens (Rue, Bitterwort) 91
Sepia (Cuttlefish ink) 91
Silicea (Silica, Pure flint,
  Rock crystal, Quartz) 92
Sulphur (Sublimated sulphur) 93
Thuja occidentalis (Arbor vitae,
  Tree of life) 94
Veratrum album (White hellebore)94
Index of Remedies 95
About This Book 96
Subject Index 96

Foreword

The word "homeopathy" is derived from Greek and means "similar suffering." Thus, the basic principle of homeopathic teaching is the Law of Similars: Let like be treated by like (*similia similibus curentur*). This means that a substance which produces certain symptoms in a healthy person will cure those same symptoms in a sick person.

The following example illustrates how this works. Imagine you have a bright red and shining face. Your pupils are dilated, and you are sweating all over, too hot in bed but freezing when uncovered. In addition, you are extremely thirsty, and your carotid artery is pulsating visibly. Your mucous membranes are bright red at first, then become dark red and patchy. Your pulse is throbbing hard and fast, and your temperature is rising.

All these symptoms occur when a healthy person eats Deadly nightshade (*Atropa belladonna*). When the symptoms are not treated, the patient normally dies. However, given in a homeopathic dosage in accordance with the Law of Similars, *Belladonna* works as a remedy for a feverish cold.

Remedies for Your Homeopathic Medicine Chest

With this self-help book you can establish the foundation of your personal homeopathic medicine chest. You can equip yourself with the complete set of medicines in the indicated potencies and be prepared for nearly all problems. Of course, you can also wait to buy the remedies until you need them. Ask a pharmacist who is knowledgeable about homeopathic remedies for advice.

For each ailment, we have selected only those remedies which we believe are the most important and the most frequently used.

> In homeopathy, an illness is treated holistically. This means that the treatment is not aimed at a symptom or ailment but at the person as a whole.

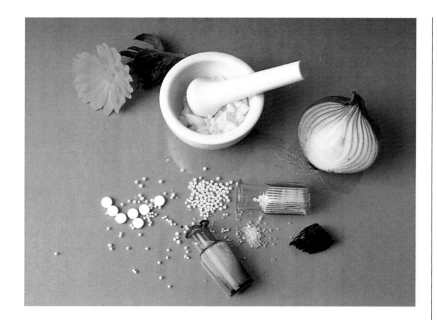

Homeopathic medicines are produced from natural materials. They are available as tablets, granules, and drops.

However, for each set of symptoms, at least a dozen other medicines could be considered useful.

Important Background Knowledge

This book not only explains how you can cure yourself effectively, it also explains what to look for so that you will be able to select the right homeopathic remedy. This basic knowledge will also be useful in communicating with your homeopathic doctor or practitioner.

Various small medicine boxes are available. Ask your homeopathic pharmacist for details.

We recommend that you go through this book so that you will know your way around it quickly when you need it. For easier access, we have listed the ailments in alphabetical order. At the end of the book, we've included an index of complaints and an index of remedies.

Michael Helfferich/Walther Hohenester

The Healing Principles of Homeopathy

Self-Healing Powers Are Activated

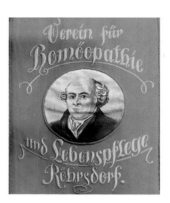

The physician and founder of homeopathy, Samuel Hahnemann, was born in 1755 in Germany. He died in 1843 in Paris.

Homeopathy is based on the principle of similarity. The correct homeopathic remedy activates the body's own self-healing powers. This concept is based on the following principles:
- Weak stimuli arouse the body's vitality.
- Medium stimuli slow down the body's vitality.
- Strong or very strong stimuli negate the body's vitality.

The Homeopathic Examination

The basis of a homeopathic treatment is a thorough examination. While laboratory results, blood pressure, and X rays are important to the homeopath, they only serve to support his or her diagnosis. The examination assesses not only the patient's symptoms but also many factors of the patient's personality.

A careful homeopathic recording of the case history takes an hour or more and includes the patient's appearance, manner of speaking, etc.

A homeopathic doctor or practitioner does not just treat the cold, headache, or diarrhea; the doctor deals with the overall symptoms the patient is experiencing. That is why there are so many different remedies for a cough or a cold: the individual cough or cold also has various symptoms.

For this reason, the same homeopathic remedy can be used to treat different diseases that have similar symptoms.

Homeopathic drugs activate the vitality of the organism so that the body can heal itself.

Samuel Hahnemann

The founder of homeopathy was Samuel Hahnemann. He established its principle, the theory of similarity, and he made countless experiments on himself. Hahnemann wrote scientific works on homeopathy which are still valid today. He worked as a homeopathic doctor until his death in 1843. It was Samuel Hahnemann who discovered the phenomenon of potentization. On finding that the mother tinctures he used caused far too strong a reaction in his patients, he began to dilute them. In doing so, he discovered that the more he diluted these remedies, the greater the effect. Hahnemann had to find a new name for this process, and he created the concept of potentization, which means making a natural substance more effective.

Hahnemann found that like is cured with like. The more he diluted, or potentized, his mother tinctures, the greater the healing effect.

Principles of Homeopathy

Law of Similars

This describes the principle of how to find the suitable medicine: like is cured with like. A medicine is given in a potentized dose which, if taken in a more concentrated dose, would cause symptoms in a healthy person.

Simile

This denotes the specific medicine that, for a given set of symptoms, stimulates the body's vitality.

Mother Tincture

Homeopathic drugs are made from a mother tincture. The component parts are derived from plants, animals, minerals, and pathogens.

Potencies

The mother tincture is diluted and shaken in specific steps (potencies).

Granules

These are sugar pellets on which the medicine is applied.

The Potencies

In the beginning, Hahnemann diluted his mother tinctures in steps of one hundred, or centesimal, potencies; later on, in the latter part of his life, he went on to develop and use LM potencies. Every homeopathic remedy exists in centesimal (C), decimal (X or D), or LM potency. These potencies simply denote the degree of dilution.

Centesimal Potencies

Only centesimal and LM potencies go back to Samuel Hahnemann. LM potencies are also called Q potencies (from the Latin *quinquaginta mila*) by some manufacturers, but this name has not been generally accepted.

■ One part of the mother substance is mixed with ninety-nine parts of alcohol and shaken vigorously one hundred times. This produces the centesimal potency 1C.

■ One part of 1C mixed together with ninety-nine parts of alcohol is shaken vigorously one hundred times to produce the potency 2C, and so forth.

■ The dilution may continue until 200C or even higher potencies are reached.

LM Potencies

LM stands for a dilution of 1 to 50,000. Granules are soaked in a drop of the relevant solution, dissolved, and soaked again.

Thus, LM6 means that a basic potency 3C is diluted in six sequences of 50,000. This is the basic method for creating LM potencies.

Decimal Potencies

This method of production was introduced in the 1930s by German physicians. To produce decimal potencies, one drop of the mother tincture is mixed with nine parts of alcohol while being vigorously shaken ten times. This is the way the first decimal potency, 1X, is prepared. The potency is then diluted with ten parts of alcohol and shaken ten times to produce 2X. You can repeat the process of sequential dilution as often as you like.

It is difficult to make general statements about the various dosages because homeopathic remedies work differently for each patient. However, the following are generally accepted.

■ Centesimal potencies take effect quickly.

■ LM potencies take effect more gently.

■ Low potencies of 4X to 6X can be used more often. For example, you can use 5–7 drops or granules two to three times a day. With children, a dosage of 4 granules two to three times a day is sufficient.

■ In acute conditions, the dose can be administered every fifteen to thirty minutes until the patient improves. Then you reduce the frequency to three times a day and, later, to one dose a day.

You must administer low potencies more frequently. The more acute an illness is, the sooner you must repeat the appropriate remedy. Please note the indicated dosage and how often you should repeat it.

Criticism of Homeopathy

With a certain grade of dilution or trituration, not a single atom of the original substance can be detected, at least not with today's methods. How then, the critics ask, can a remedy have any effect at all? What they overlook is the decisive process of succussion. Theories explaining the release of energy by the procedure of potentizing have existed for some time. The quantum theory has brought us a large step closer to understanding this mystery.

Nevertheless, to this point, scientists have no conclusive explanation of how, for instance, a high centesimal potency can take effect. However, the successful cures brought about daily through homeopathy show that such an effect really does exist.

When you take into account not only the symptoms but also the accompanying circumstances, you'll find the right remedy more easily.

Taking too high or too low a potency or taking a medicine too often can aggravate the symptoms or can cancel out the desired effect. You can avoid such unintentional effects by using the potencies indicated and taking them in the recommended way.

Finding the Right Remedy

Homeopathy primarily observes the physical, mental, and emotional symptoms of an illness:

- How long has the illness lasted?
- Where do the complaints arise?
- How do the symptoms manifest themselves?
- What alleviates or aggravates the condition? (These are the modalities.)
- In what way has the general state of health changed?
- What else is there that seems unusual or peculiar? (A patient's likes and dislikes.)

The Modalities

The question of aggravating or alleviating an ailment is of particular importance. This is what is meant by the term "modalities": What makes the condition better or worse? When? In what frame of mind?

Example: A case of diarrhea and vomiting is worse with cold, in cold and wet weather, and after midnight; but it improves with warmth and warm drinks. These modalities clearly point to *Arsenicum album* (Arsenic trioxide, White arsenic).

The Right Dosage

Please use the selected remedy in the dosage recommended by us! As a general rule, in acute cases, you can give a remedy every fifteen to thirty minutes until you notice improvement. Then, reduce the dosage to three times a day and, finally, to once a day. The correct way to take homeopathic medicine is to put the granules under your tongue ten minutes before a meal (one to three times a day) and to let them dissolve slowly. Before taking the medicine, you should rinse your mouth with water.

How to Take the Medicine

In the following pages we have provided the exact dosage of every homeopathic remedy described. This is normally given in the form of granules.

In the case of acute complaints, if you observe no improvement whatsoever after three doses (in the case of chronic complaints, after one week), stop taking the medicine. You can try one or two other remedies in the recommended dosage or consult an experienced homeopath. If your symptoms do not go away completely with the applied medicine, take five granules of the same medicine in the potency 12C once a day for three to five days. If in doubt, consult your family doctor, pharmacist, or an experienced homeopath. Important: If acute symptoms persist for longer than twenty-four hours or if they worsen, consult your health care practitioner.

Constitutional Medicine

A homeopath does not treat an illness; he or she treats the person who is ill. Before beginning a treatment, the homeopath observes all of the patient's symptoms. The kind of pain described by the patient is just as important to the homeopath as the person's clothing, way of speaking, and reaction to outside influences.

Constitutional medicine is the remedy that best corresponds with the entirety of a person's physical, mental, and emotional symptoms.

A patient can, for instance, be an *Arsenicum album* type, a *Pulsatilla* type, or a *Sepia* type, depending on which homeopathic remedy, *Arsenicum*, *Pulsatilla*, or *Sepia*, is most similar to the patient's overall appearance. (See "The 31 Most Important Remedies," beginning on page 81).

> To a homeopath, a constitutional medicine is a medicine that corresponds not only to a patient's complaints but also to his or her main character traits.

Ailments from A to Z

Abdominal Pain

Abdominal pain can be a symptom of many ailments. Gallstones, diseases of the kidneys, or appendicitis can be responsible. Small children respond to many different illnesses by complaining of a stomachache.

Nux vomica (Poison nut)

Use *Nux vomica* for convulsive abdominal pain after a disappointment, irritation, or anger; drug abuse (painkillers or laxatives); excessive consumption of alcohol, nicotine, or coffee; heavy meals; or eating spoiled food. The patient complains of a feeling of fullness, flatulence in the upper abdomen, heartburn, and constipation. The stomachache begins about an hour after a meal. The condition is worse in the mornings. Heavy food, alcohol, and anger also have negative effects. The condition improves with warmth, warm compresses, and rest.

- Dosage: 3 granules of *Nux vomica* 6C every hour; after improvement, 5 granules twice a day

Magnesium phosphoricum (Magnesium phosphate)

Use for all kinds of spasmodic pains. The pains are worse when cold, when touched, and during menstruation. The symptoms improve by pressing, by doubling up, by applying a hot-water bottle, or by massaging the painful areas.

- Dosage: 3 granules of *Magnesium phosphoricum* 12C every hour; after improvement, 5 granules once or twice a day

Colocynthis (Bitter cucumber)

Colocynthis helps relieve gripping pains in the stomach and abdomen after irritation and anger. These pains feel as if sharp

If you have very severe or recurring abdominal attacks, you should discuss the cause with your doctor or practitioner.

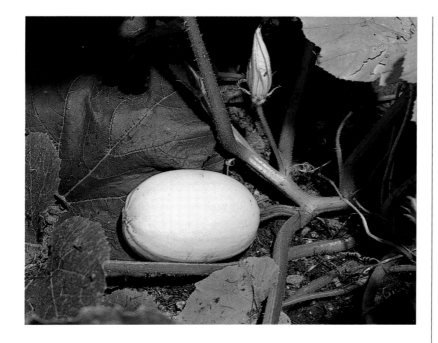

Citrullus colocynthis *(Bitter cucumber)* belongs to the squash family. The homeopathic medicine Colocynthis *is prepared from the ripe, peeled, and cored fruit.*

stones were rubbing against each other. The patient is uneasy, irritable, restless, and annoyed. The complaints increase after meals, after eating fruit, and before and during menstruation. The patient feels better by doubling up, leaning forward and drawing his or her legs up, as well as by applying warmth, by pressing hard against the painful area, by passing gas, and by passing stool.

■ Dosage: 3 granules of *Colocynthus* 6C every hour; then 5 granules twice a day

Magnesium phosphoricum can also be used as the "Hot Seven" (Dr. Schuessler's functional remedy): Dissolve 10 tablets of *Magnesium phosphoricum* 6x in 8 ounces (250ml) of hot water and sip it every fifteen minutes until the pain is completely gone.

Abscess, Suppuration

The danger of abscesses and suppuration is that they may spread or that the organism which produces the pus may enter the bloodstream and the lymphatic system, causing blood poisoning. The patient does best when the pus can drain out of the body. The abscess may have to be surgically cut, or the patient may use one of the following homeopathic remedies. To help the treatment, apply a compress of clay with healing properties and a poultice or drawing ointment.

Myristica sebifera (Bark of the ucuuba tree)

We call this medicine the "homeopathic knife." *Myristica sebifera* accelerates the body's defensive process so that the abscess opens, and the pus flows out.

- Dosage: 5 granules of *Myristica sebifera* 3C every half hour; then 5 granules three times a day after the abscess has opened

Belladonna (Deadly nightshade)

Use *Belladonna* if the skin around the abscess is dark red, very swollen, and hot. The patient complains of severe, often throbbing pain. The abscess is extremely sensitive to touch and to pressure. The symptoms are accompanied by headaches, and the patient is irritable and aggressive.

- Dosage: 3 granules of *Belladonna* 6C every half hour; after improvement, 5 granules (maximum) three times a day

Hepar sulphuris (Calcium sulphide)

Hepar sulphuris helps with injuries that tend to suppurate. The suppurating wounds or abscesses are extremely painful and sensitive to touch, and the patient sweats and has sharp pains. Cold or pressure makes the condition worse. Warm compresses improve the patient's condition.

- Dosage: 1 tablet of *Hepar sulphuris* 4C every hour; after the pus has begun to flow, 1 tablet three times a day or 3 granules of 12C every hour; after improvement, 3 granules three times a day

The homeopathic medicine Silicea *is produced from rock crystal.*

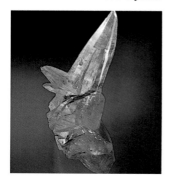

Silicea (Quartz)

Silicea helps patients with sensitive, fine, and pale skin who have a tendency to prolonged suppuration. It is effective with suppuration after a cut caused by glass. Suppurating infections of the nail bed also respond to *Silicea*.

■ Dosage: 1 tablet of *Silicea* 4C every hour; then 1 tablet three times a day; or 3 granules 12C every hour, then 3 granules three times a day

Acne

Acne is an inflammatory disease of the hair follicles and sebaceous glands. In most cases, it is caused by poorly functioning intestines or digestive organs or by a hormonal imbalance. As a general measure, we recommend eating raw fruit and vegetables rich in vitamins, dry brushing the skin, and avoiding sugar, sweets, alcohol, and nicotine.

Some good basic treatments are available as acne capsules, acne face lotions, acne steam baths, and acne face masks. You can find these products at selected health food stores.

Selenium (Selenium)
Selenium is a good remedy for teenage acne, which is characterized by very oily skin with lots of little itchy pimples or blackheads. Dry, flaking rashes on the palms and an itching in the finger joints and between the fingers are also typical symptoms. The condition worsens before and during menstruation.
■ Dosage: 5 granules of *Selenium* 12C once a day

Silicea (Quartz)
Silicea helps with pimples, blackheads, and boils that tend to become inflamed and then suppurate. Acne pimples are often hard and leave scars. The patient's nails may be thick and deformed.

Wholesome Food to Help Fight Acne
■ Lots of fresh fruit and vegetables.
■ Whole grain products.
■ Milk and milk products.
■ Herbal teas with horsetail, dandelion, and stinging nettle.

They break off easily or have white spots.

■ Dosage: 5 granules of *Silicea* 12C once a day

Kali bromatum (Bromide of potash, Potassium bromide)

You can use *Kali bromatum* to treat brownish, hard, and itching pimples on the face, breast, and shoulders that ooze a creamlike secretion when scratched. Additional symptoms are a dazed and restless feeling, especially in the hands. *Kali bromatum* and lichens also help with severe itching that often spreads all over the body. The acne gets worse during menstruation or in a warm bed.

■ Dosage: 5 granules of *Kali bromatum* 6C once a day

Juglans regia (Walnut)

Juglans regia relieves common acne of the face, shoulders, and back. The skin often itches and tingles when hot. Scratching aggravates the acne.

■ Dosage: 5 granules of *Juglans regia* 3C twice a day

Sulphur iodatum (Iodide of sulphur)

Sulphur iodatum has proved successful with teenage acne that has developed into suppurating lumps. Characteristically, the affected parts have a dark red border. You can also use this remedy for impetigo that has suppurating lumps and red patches. Another typical symptom is that the patient does not gain weight despite having a large appetite.

■ Dosage: 5 granules of *Sulphur iodatum* 6C once a day

Hepar sulphuris (Calcium sulphide)

Adolescents who have severe acne in which the pustules with white pus sting painfully and who have dry skin respond well to *Hepar sulphuris*. These patients frequently catch colds after the weather turns cold or from drafts and are susceptible to sore throats from cold air or cold drinks. They are discontented and become irritated quickly.

■ Dosage: 5 granules of *Hepar sulphuris* 12C once a day

Never squeeze pimples or blackheads. An experienced practitioner should do this, otherwise there is the danger of a secondary infection that can leave ugly scars.

Appetite Disorders

Most people find that their appetite is a barometer for their basic physical and emotional condition. Physical ailments, strain, overexertion, grief, worry, and depression are noticeable because of changes in the appetite.

Appetite Disorders—Excessive Appetite

Solanum tuberosum (Potato berries)
We refer to this remedy as an herbal appetite suppressant.
- Dosage: 10 granules of *Solanum tuberosum* 3C three times a day

Lycopodium (Club moss)
In the afternoons and at night, ravenous hunger prevents sleep. *Lycopodium* is also helpful in treating excessive appetite accompanied by stomachache. The craving for food can recur shortly after the meal and then subside after a few bites, or it may increase with eating.
- Dosage: 5 granules of *Lycopodium* 6C twice a day

Calcium carbonicum (Calcium carbonate)
Calcium carbonicum is the appropriate remedy if ravenous hunger is due to a constant empty feeling in the stomach that persists even after eating, such as with diarrhea. There is usually a craving for sweets, ice cream, and eggs and a desire for or an aversion to milk.
- Dosage: 3 granules of *Calcium carbonicum* 12C twice a day

With appetite problems, the most important way to support the homeopathic medicine is to find the cause of the problem.

Cravings during pregnancy

Try not to surrender to cravings for sweets because sugary foods interfere with the development of the fetus's teeth and bones. Spoil yourself in other ways. For instance, go for a walk, have a massage, listen to music, or enjoy a good conversation.

Appetite Disorders—Loss of Appetite

China (Peruvian bark)

After a severe illness or a loss of blood and body fluids, patients may lose their appetite, even though they are hungry, because they have a sensation of fullness. If patients can bring themselves to eat, their appetite usually returns after the first few bites. *China* 6C helps relieve a loss of appetite in foggy weather.
- Dosage: 5 granules of *China* 6C twice a day

Sulphur (Sublimated sulphur)

The appetite disappears at the sight of food, but the person is very thirsty.
- Dosage: 5 granules of *Sulphur* 6C twice a day

Ignatia (St. Ignatius bean)

When people are emotionally unhappy or disappointed, they may experience a loss of appetite, usually in the daytime. At night they are so hungry that they cannot fall asleep. They feel an aversion to food and do not like anything. This feeling is stronger during menstruation.
- Dosage: 5 granules of *Ignatia* 6C twice a day

Backache

Injuries to the spinal nerves are painful, but we can relieve or cure them with homeopathic remedies. In addition, compresses with

If a lack of appetite or an excess of appetite continues over a long period, consider the possibility of a worm disorder, especially in children. Your doctor or homeopath will be able to help you.

alcoholic liniment and St. John's-wort oil are effective, as are massages and, in some cases, heat treatment.

■ Dosage: 5 granules 6C of the indicated remedy twice a day; on improvement, 5 granules once a day

Arnica (Leopard's bane)

Weariness and a fear of being touched are typical symptoms suggesting the use of *Arnica*. The bed seems too hard, and the patient wants to be left alone. The symptoms are worse with movement and touch and in cold, wet weather. They improve when resting.

Apis mellifica (Honeybee)

A treatment with *Apis* relieves rheumatic backache with burning and shooting pains. Cold compresses also improve the symptoms.

Rhus toxicodendron (Poison Ivy)

Rhus toxicodendron is the remedy for strains accompanied by a feeling of numbness and paralysis in the legs. The symptoms are worse when resting, at night, and in moist or wet weather. They improve with warmth, rubbing, and continued movement.

Bellis perennis (Daisy)

If the nerves are affected after a back injury, take *Bellis perennis*. The symptoms are aggravated by touch and by the warmth of bed and hot baths. Cold baths do not provide relief. The symptoms improve with a constant, even motion.

Prolonged or recurrent backache could be an indication of electromagnetic fields in the sleeping area or of unsuitable materials in the mattress and pillow.

Learn how to protect your back against pain and illness. Be sure to exercise carefully.

Support for Your Back
■ Remember to sit in an upright position.
■ Do not carry heavy loads on one side.
■ Always lift heavy loads from a squatting position.
■ Wear comfortable shoes; never wear high heels.
■ Exercise your back muscles regularly.

Conium (Poison hemlock)

Use *Conium* when a spinal injury is accompanied by giddiness, sickness, and numbness in the lower half of the body. You can also use this remedy for neuralgia of the coccyx that is worse when standing. The symptoms are worse when the patient is bumped or jarred, and they improve with movement.

■ Dosage: Always consult a homeopath!

Bladder and Kidney Inflammation

With bladder problems, it is often difficult even for the experienced homeopath to find the correct remedy. The following medicines are those that we believe are the most important. In addition, we strongly recommend warm or rising footbaths. Be sure to keep your feet and legs warm.

■ Dosage: 5 granules of the indicated remedy in the potency 6C three times a day; after improvement of the symptoms, twice a day for a few more days; and then once a day

If the pain becomes worse, you have a high temperature, or the symptoms migrate up to the kidneys, see a doctor or an experienced homeopath immediately.

Apis mellifica (Honeybee)

Apis mellifica is a suitable remedy for cystitis with a persistent urge to urinate but with little or no discharge of urine. Stinging and burning pain occurs while urinating, and the pain increases with the last drops. The urethra is sore and feels scalded. The dark urine contains a lot of protein and sediment. Edema (an accumulation of fluid) develops in the arms and legs and on the eyelids. In the afternoons, the patient often runs a high temperature with shivering. He or she is thirsty (except when running a fever) and sleepy.

Cantharis (Spanish fly)

With cystitis that is contracted after sunburn, there is a constant, violent urge to urinate, along with spasms in the bladder often accompanied by backache. The urine is frequently dark red and only comes in drops. These cause a burning or cutting pain in the

Preventing Cystitis

As a preventive measure, take rising footbaths:

- Fill a bucket with warm water at about 90° F (32°C).
- Step into the bucket with both legs.
- Add hot water every minute for ten minutes, so that the temperature rises by about 1.5°F (1° C) a minute to about 105° F (42°C).
- Keep the water temperature at 105° F (42°C) for another ten minutes.
- After a rising footbath, lie down and rest for about fifteen minutes.

urethra. The pain persists before, during, and after urination. *Cantharis* is the remedy for this, as well as for pyelitis with sensitivity to the lightest touch. Often the patient runs a high temperature, has cold hands and feet, has a cold sweat, is very restless, and is constantly thirsty. The condition is worse after drinking and on touching, but it improves after applications of heat.

Dulcamara (Bittersweet)

Dulcamara has proved to be an effective remedy against cystitis that follows catching cold, getting wet, wearing a wet bathing suit, changing weather, and sitting on a cold surface. The urethra hurts while urinating. The urine is cloudy, salty, slimy, and foul smelling. Damp cold aggravates the condition.

Lycopodium (Club moss)

Lycopodium is effective against catarrh of the bladder and the pelvis of the kidney. It is also the main remedy for kidney stones. The patient experiences a painful burning during and after urination. After efforts to press, the urine usually flows slowly with a pungent smell and red sediment. Children cry before urinating. The backache that occurs before urinating disappears afterwards.

Pulsatilla (Wind flower) is appropriate for cystitis caused by a chill, by allowing your feet to get cold, or during pregnancy. Cystitis is accompanied by a constant urge to urinate that is worse when lying down. Additional symptoms include a burning pain after urinating, an involuntary discharge of urine when sneezing, coughing, or laughing, and flatulence. Continued movement improves the symptoms.

Take *Berberis* (Barberry) if you frequently have to urinate urgently, experience burning and cutting pains in the urethra (especially before and during urinating), and have pain in the thighs and hips while urinating. The urine continually changes its appearance and contains a light red or yellow sediment and a thick slime. Movement and bumping aggravate the condition. Resting improves it.

Bad Breath

Persistent bad breath is an irksome and often repulsive problem. Medicinal mouthwashes and chewing gum usually provide only temporary help.

■ Dosage: 5 granules 6C of the indicated remedy twice a day

Pulsatilla (Wind flower)

Foul-smelling or putrid breath develops (especially in the morning) after eating fatty food or pastry. The mouth is dry, but the patient is not thirsty. The tongue is yellow or white and covered with thick saliva.

Nux vomica (Poison nut)

Nux vomica helps relieve putrid, sour, or foul-smelling breath that occurs especially in the mornings after heavy evening meals. The bad breath gets worse with eating. The person usually exhibits general irritability.

Teucrium (Cat thyme)

This remedy improves musty breath caused by mucus in the throat in cases of chronic sinusitis.

Sinapis nigra (Black mustard)

Sinapis nigra helps when the breath smells of onions or garlic.

Taraxacum (Dandelion)

The person has a taste of feces in his mouth due to a weak liver. A white film covers the tongue. It comes off in pieces leaving red, sensitive spots on the tongue.

Burns

You can treat a minor burn by putting it under cold running water and then cleansing the wound with undiluted vinegar (not vinegar concentrate) or with *Calendula* mother tincture: 10 drops to one

Bad breath can be an indication of an internal disease, such as gastritis, ulcers, and other intestinal diseases. It can also point to a zinc deficiency, periodontal problems, and tooth decay.

Cedron (Rattlesnake bean) is the remedy for putrid or foul-smelling breath during menstruation.

If *Taraxacum* (Dandelion) does not relieve the feeling of constantly having bad breath, try *Chelidonium* (Celandine). This is a remedy for stomach and liver complaints that are relieved by hot food and warm drinks.

glass of boiled and cooled water. Then apply a dressing with Combuduron gel (Weleda), which you can purchase at your homeopathic pharmacy.

Arnica (Leopard's bane)

As a first homeopathic measure, *Arnica* helps relieve the shock.
- Dosage: 5 granules of *Arnica* 6C every fifteen minutes; or 3 granules of *Arnica* 30C two to three times, an hour apart

Belladonna (Deadly nightshade)

Belladonna is effective if the skin is bright red and patchy and the patient feels a throbbing pain around the burn.
- Dosage: 3 granules of *Belladonna* 6C every fifteen minutes

Ferrum phosphoricum (Ferrum phosphate)

Use *Ferrum phosphoricum* if the skin is red and very tender to the touch.
- Dosage: 5 granules of *Ferrum phosphoricum* 12C every hour

Hamamelis (Witch hazel)

Hamamelis is a specific remedy used when you burn your tongue or lips with hot drinks.
- Dosage: 5 granules of *Hamamelis* 4C every fifteen minutes

Degrees of Burns	
Degree I:	Reddening
Degree II:	Blisters
Degree III:	Open wounds
Degree IV:	Charred skin

First Aid for Burns

- Immediately place the burn under cold running water or submerge the injured part in cold water for at least ten to twenty minutes
- Remove burned clothing, but do not pull at pieces of clothing that are sticking to the burned area.
- Never open a blister.
- Cover the burn well with dry, sterile compresses.
- With minor burns, a burn ointment provides relief.
- In cases of extensive or severe burns, you must call for an ambulance.

With minor burns, you can ease the pain by placing the burn close to the heat source again. Repeat two or three times. This is another example of like cured with like. The pain usually goes away, and blisters do not develop.

Arsenicum album (Arsenic trioxide, White arsenic)

Arsenicum album helps when there is a burning pain and blisters develop. The injured person is anxious and does not want to be left alone.

■ Dosage: 2 granules of *Arsenicum album* 12C every half hour

Urtica urens (Stinging nettle)

Use *Urtica urens* for burns with indented blisters. The patient feels a burning pain and itching. Cold, touch, and cold water make the symptoms worse.

■ Dosage: 5 granules of *Urtica urens* 6C every hour

Cantharis (Spanish fly)

Blisters develop with a burning pain. Chills alternate with hot flushes, and the patient is restless.

■ Dosage: 3 granules of *Cantharis* 6C every fifteen minutes

Third and Fourth Degree Burns

With severe burns (third and fourth degree), use homeopathic remedies as a first-aid measure to support the medical treatment.

Burns that are larger than the palm of your hand must be treated immediately by an emergency doctor.

Arsenicum album (Arsenic trioxide, White arsenic)

Give *Arsenicum album* if the borders of the blisters have become black.

■ Dosage: 3 granules of *Arsenicum album* 12C every ten minutes

Causticum (Potassium sulphate)

Use *Causticum* in cases where the skin is charred.

■ Dosage: 5 granules of *Causticum* 6C every ten minutes

Canker Sores

If canker sores or other diseases of the mucous membranes in the mouth occur occasionally, determine what metal alloys (fillings, bridges) are in the mouth. A stool examination can ascertain whether the intestines are infected with fungi or germs.

Sempervivum (House leek)

Sempervivum is a specific remedy for canker sores. Use it until the symptoms abate.

■ Dosage: 5 granules of *Sempervivum* 4C three times a day

Borax (Sodium borate)

White canker sores on the mucous membranes in the mouth and on the tongue that develop quickly and tend to bleed respond to *Borax*. Patients usually complain of a dry mouth. They may also have diarrhea.

■ Dosage: 3 granules of *Borax* 6C three times a day; after improvement, 5 granules once a day

Mercurius solubilis (Mercury)

Use *Mercurius solubilis* for bluish red inflammation of the gums and mucous membranes of the mouth, including canker sores and ulcer points. The saliva is often bloody, and the patient's breath is foul smelling. The tongue is covered with a slimy yellow-green fur, which has indentations from the teeth at the sides. The gums are spongy and very sensitive to the touch. They often bleed when touched. The teeth can become loose. The pain is worse at night and is alleviated by warmth and warm drinks.

■ Dosage: 5 granules of *Mercurius solubilis* 6C twice a day: when convalescing, once a day

Acidum nitricum (Nitric acid)

Canker sores and ulcers that tend to bleed are very painful and feel as if needles or splinters of wood have pierced the inflamed

In addition to the recommended treatment, daub with *Propolis* extract or with a tincture of *Calendula* (Marigold) diluted to 10 percent, *Tormentilla* (Tormentil), or *Hamamelis* (Witch hazel). These are available at health food stores.

Borax is often the correct remedy for stomatitis in infants.

When concentrated nitric acid comes into contact with the skin or the mucous membranes, a syndrome develops that is similar to that of canker sores. You can heal this with *Acidum nitricum*.

parts. There is profuse saliva with foul breath and a sweetish taste; the gums are mostly spongy and retract from the base of the teeth. Just sucking on them can make them bleed. You can often see a furrow along the center line of the moist, reddened tongue. The lips and the corners of the mouth are chapped.

■ Dosage: 5 granules of *Acidum nitricum* 6C twice a day; after improvement, once a day

Acidum sulphuricum (Sulfuric acid)

Canker sores and ulcers exude a dark, thin, bloody secretion. The gums tend to bleed, there is profuse saliva, and the breath is foul. Patients who suffer from these are often hasty and weak people who feel the cold and suffer from heartburn and sour burping.

■ Dosage: 5 granules of *Acidum sulphuricum* 6C twice a day

Catarrh

From the homeopathic point of view, the common catarrh is nothing more than a cleansing act of the body via the mucous membranes. If the catarrh is chronic, you should have your stool examined for intestinal parasites. It may also be wise to have an allergy test done to check for hay fever.

To increase the body's defenses, take mother tincture of *Echinacea angustifolia* (dosage: 15 drops three times a day) or *Echinacea* 3x (5 granules three times a day).

Allium cepa (Red onion)

Use *Allium cepa* for a runny nose with acrid, frequent discharge, often accompanied by a spasmodic cough and a tickling in the larynx that is caused by cold and damp weather, and by wind. The symptoms are worse in rooms with warm, humid air. They improve outdoors.

■ Dosage: 3 granules of *Allium cepa* 6C every two hours

Euphrasia (Eyebright)

The catarrh is mild, but the tears are acrid and irritate the skin. The patient sneezes a lot and is very sensitive to light. The symptoms are worse in warm rooms and in the daytime. The flow of

> **How to Strengthen the Body's Defenses**
> ∎ Avoid stimulants such as alcohol and nicotine.
> ∎ Exercise in the fresh air.
> ∎ Get enough sleep.
> ∎ Go to a sauna often.
> ∎ Eat plenty of fresh fruit and vegetables.
> ∎ If possible, do not eat pork.
> ∎ Apply cold affusions.

tears increases in the cold and wind. This improves when the patient is lying down.

∎ Dosage: 3 granules of *Euphrasia* 6C every two hours.

Luffa (Sponge gourd)

Take *Luffa* if a flowing or stuffy nose is accompanied by tiredness and if a dull headache radiates from the forehead to the back of the neck.

∎ Dosage: 5 granules of *Luffa* 4C three times a day

Sambucus (Elder)

Use *Sambucus* when the nose is blocked but there is no discharge. Breathing difficulty is possible at night when the inflammation extends to the throat. Try warm throat compresses. The symptoms are worse at night, in warm temperatures, and in dry air.

∎ Dosage: 5 granules of *Sambucus* 6C every two to three hours

Pulsatilla (Wind flower)

An alternate way to treat a stuffy and runny nose. The symptoms are worse in the evening when lying down. They improve in fresh air and with exercise.

∎ Dosage: 5 granules of *Pulsatilla* 6C every two to three hours

You can also use the homeopathic remedies for catarrh when you have hay fever accompanied by the symptoms described above.

A catarrh is not just a troublesome disease of the nose. It serves as a means of cleansing and regenerating the whole body. Because it is the body's defensive reaction against invading germs, you should not try to suppress catarrh with chemical agents.

■ *Vincetoxicum* (Swallow wort) enhances the body's defenses against viral coughs and sneezes. Take it as a preventive or at the onset of the condition. Dosage: 5 granules 3C three times a day.

■ The combination of *Vincetoxicum* 3C and *Sulphur* 6C has a positive effect on the immune system. Dosage: 5 granules of each remedy three times a day.

Arsenicum album (Arsenic trioxide, White arsenic)

If the discharge is thin, watery, and acrid, *Arsenicum album* is good for apprehensive patients who are very thirsty and who frequently drink small amounts of liquid. The symptoms are worse in the cold. They improve with warmth.

■ Dosage: 3 granules of *Arsenicum album* 12C twice a day

Colds

In case of colds, see the entries for "Catarrh," "Cough," "Earache," "Fever," "Flu-like Symptoms," and "Sore Throat." To prevent a cold, or at the onset of a cold, we recommend a light diet rich in vitamins in addition to the following remedies.

Echinacea angustifolia (Cone flower)

The patient feels weak and exhausted, as if he has been ill for a long time. He has a strong sensation of being chilled. At the onset of the cold, the patient asks impatiently when he is going to get better. He aches all over and is susceptible to a weak heart and to collapsing. Eating causes fermentation and bloating in the stomach. There is often sour burping and heartburn.

■ Dosage: 5 granules of *Echinacea angustifolia* 3C three times a day

Conjunctivitis

Conjunctivitis can arise on its own or in conjunction with a general illness.

Belladonna (Deadly nightshade)

Belladonna helps if the conjunctivitis is due to looking at a bright light (glacier, welding, etc.), to cold and wet weather, or to a draft. The conjunctiva is bright red and swollen, and the pupils are dilated. The eye usually remains dry and is very sensitive to light.

■ Dosage: 3 granules of *Belladonna* 6C three times a day

Euphrasia (Eyebright)

Euphrasia is the appropriate remedy if conjunctivitis is due to wind or occurs along with a cold or hay fever. Typically, there is an acrid flow of tears. Sometimes there is suppuration, and the conjunctiva looks red and swollen. The tears feel hot, and the eye blinks almost uncontrollably. The condition is aggravated by light (sunlight or artificial light), reading, writing, cold, wind, and by warm rooms. The symptoms improve in the dark or by blinking.

■ Dosage: 3 granules of *Euphrasia* 6C three times a day

Pulsatilla (Wind flower)

Pulsatilla is the correct remedy if tears flow with an abundant yellowish or suppurating secretion after exposure to wind, cold air, or with a cold. The eyelids are red, swollen, and stuck together when the patient wakes up in the morning, but there is no pain. When you have dryness with a sandy feeling and a strong urge to rub your eyes, the symptoms often respond to *Pulsatilla*. The condition is worse in warm rooms. It improves in the fresh air or with cold compresses applied to the eye. You can also treat sties with *Pulsatilla*.

■ Dosage: 5 granules of *Pulsatilla* 6C once or twice a day

Ruta graveolens (Bitter rue)

Use *Ruta* to treat redness and burning of the eyes, a feeling of heat, and a headache that occurs after you have strained your eyes. Typical symptoms are a constant desire to rub the eyes and difficulty adjusting the eyes to different distances.

■ Dosage: 5 granules of *Ruta* 6C once or twice a day

Sepia (Cuttlefish ink)

Sepia is an important remedy for conjunctivitis with dry eyes in the evenings, which occurs in the spring. The eyelids are red, scaly, and sometimes sagging. The remedy has also been successful in treating diminished eyesight that occurs in conjunction with diseases of the uterus. The symptoms are aggravated in the morn-

For conjunctivitis, apply the following eye drops: With severe redness, apply *Euphrasia* (Eyebright) 3x; with redness and suppuration of the eyes, use an *Echinacea* (Quartz) compound, putting 1 drop in each eye three times a day.

Note the expiration date before you use eye drops and never use a bottle that someone else has used. Do not share eye drops with other people and do not touch your eyes with the dropper.

If a foreign body enters the eye, immediately try to rinse it out with cold running water. If this does not work, you must see an eye specialist.

ings and evenings or in hot weather. A cold bath improves the condition.

■ Dosage: 3 granules of *Sepia* 12C twice a day

Aconite (Monk's hood)

Aconite will help if conjunctivitis occurs with severe pain after exposure to dry weather or cold wind, after injuries, or from foreign bodies in the eye (sand, earth, etc.). The eye is dry and red, and the patient has a sensation of heat and sand in the eye.

■ Dosage: 5 granules of *Aconite* 6C every 2 to three hours until the condition improves

Apis (Honeybee)

Use *Apis* for suppurating inflammations with a strong, glassy swelling of the eyelids, burning, stinging, and hot tears.

■ Dosage: 3 granules of *Apis* 6C three times a day

Ferrum phosphoricum (Ferrum phosphate)

Ferrum phosphoricum is the appropriate treatment with acute catarrhs accompanied by a burning dryness and red inflammation of the eye but with no secretion of mucus or pus. Moving the eye aggravates the condition.

■ Dosage: 5 granules of *Ferrum phosphoricum* 12C twice a day

If conjunctivitis becomes chronic, you should see your eye specialist. He can also ascertain whether the irritation has any connection with a visual defect.

Rhus toxicodendron (Poison ivy)

Rhus toxicodendron is appropriate for conjunctivitis caused by allowing the eyes to become wet or as a result of cold and wet weather. The eyelids are swollen, stuck together, and suppurating in the morning. Once the eyes are open, a torrent of hot tears flows, and the skin turns red or pimply in the places touched by the tears. The eyes are extremely sensitive to light, even at night.

■ Dosage: 5 granules of *Rhus toxicodendron* 6C twice a day

Natrium muriaticum (Sodium chloride, Table salt)

If wind is the cause of the flow of tears in conjunctivitis, use

Natrium muriaticum. Additional symptoms are an inflamed eyelid with a sandy feeling in the morning, a discharge of mucus and pus when pressing on the lachrymal sack, pressure in the eye or headaches, and eye strain, sensitivity to light, letters running together while reading, and tears streaming down the face when coughing or laughing. Wind makes the condition worse.

■ Dosage: 5 granules of *Natrium muriaticum* 6C twice a day.

Thuja occidentalis (Arbor vitae, Tree of life)

Thuja is the appropriate remedy for inflammation of the eyelid and conjunctiva with swelling, tearing eyes, and sensitivity to light. Painless blisters appear on the conjunctiva and cornea. The patient has a sensation of a cold draft blowing across the eyes. The eyesight may be dimmed, and the field of vision may be reduced.

■ Dosage: 5 granules of *Thuja* 6C twice a day

If you have conjunctivitis, protect your eyes from wind, cold air, dust, etc. Intense weeping may lead to an improvement of the complaint, due to the cleansing power of the tears. Sometimes this cures the condition completely.

Constipation

Eating meals that have little or no roughage, a lack of exercise, and nervousness are only a few of the causes of troublesome constipation. It is also frequently a disagreeable travel companion. Homeopathy offers quite a number of possibilities for curing constipation.

Bryonia (White hops, White bryony)

The dry stool is large and hard. Typically, the patient is thirsty and drinks large amounts of cold water.

■ Dosage: 5 granules of *Bryonia* 6C twice a day

If possible do not take laxatives. Taken over a long period of time, they only aggravate the problem.

Alumen (Potash alum)

Alumen is the best remedy if you have the feeling your anus is contracting from hard, large stools.

■ Dosage: 5 Granules of *Alumen* 6C twice a day

Use *China* if constipation occurs after a loss of fluids, such as after profuse sweating or diarrhea. *China* can also be helpful in constipation after a loss of blood or after pregnancy and birth. Dosage: 5 granules *China* 6C twice a day.

The Correct Diet with Constipation

■ Eat unprocessed foods rich in roughage.

■ Drink at least five or six pints of liquid a day.

■ Eat linseed or bran mixed with yogurt or similar milk product.

■ Every morning, eat one or two prunes that have soaked overnight in a little water.

Plumbum metallicum (Lead)

Treat with *Plumbum metallicum* when the sphincter cramps and evacuation of the bowels is painful and often only possible with hard straining.

■ Dosage: 3 granules of *Plumbum metallicum* 12C twice a day

Lycopodium (Club moss)

Constipation often occurs when you have to use public rest rooms. In addition, you may suffer from flatulence in the lower abdomen.

■ Dosage: 5 granules of *Lycopodium* 6C twice a day

Nux vomica (Poison nut)

Nervous constipation usually occurs when people are traveling. It is very stubborn, although the bowel movement seems to be quite normal. The patient is angry, and this anger makes the constipation worse.

■ Dosage: 5 granules of *Nux vomica* 6C twice a day

Bronchitis Cough

Coughs usually come along with colds. Thus, the first thing you should do is to fortify your body by giving it rest, warmth, and suitable nourishment. In addition to the homeopathic treatment, you can relieve your lungs with herbal teas and chest compresses.

Belladonna (Deadly nightshade)

Coughs can occur in cold, dry weather or in times of great tension in the family. The dry, barking, sometimes spasmodic cough begins suddenly and violently. A tickling or scraping in the throat triggers the cough. Children suddenly awake from sleep and cry before, during, or after coughing. Stomachache or headache, especially in the forehead, may accompany coughing. The condition is worse at night, during sleep, when speaking, and with cold.

■ Dosage: Begin with 5 granules of *Belladonna* 6C every hour; with improvement, increase the intervals

Hepar sulphuris (Calcium sulphide)

Bronchial complaints occur after a fairly long exposure to dry cold or with suppressed skin eruptions. The cough is dry and spasmodic but rarely rattling. It is triggered by the sensation of a splinter between the larynx and the bronchi. Children cry at night before, during, or after a fit of coughing. The coughs and the pains increase gradually. The patient may be extremely sensitive to cold. The condition is worse at night and on waking in the morning. The slightest exposure to cold or even cold drinks can trigger the cough. Damp, warm air, humidifiers, steam baths, and inhaling steam improve the condition.

■ Dosage: 3 granules of *Hepar sulphuris* 12C every two hours; increase the intervals with improvement

Bryonia (Wild hops, White bryony)

Dry cough with shooting pains behind the breastbone increases gradually until it becomes unbearable. It occurs in the fall. Pressing hard against the painful region eases the shooting pains. The patient is moody and irritable and only wants to be left alone. He is very thirsty. Entering a warm room, breathing deeply, and speaking worsen the condition. The symptoms are improved by drinking warm fluids, remaining motionless, or keeping a firm hold of the thorax.

■ Dosage: 5 granules of *Bryonia* 6C every two hours

We advise you not to use ethereal oils or other substances with strong odors for inhalation or for massage because we cannot be sure whether these strong odors cancel out the effect of certain homeopathic remedies.

Bryonia alba *(Wild hops, White bryony). The medicine extracted from these plants is helpful for rheumatic pain and complaints of the mucous membranes.*

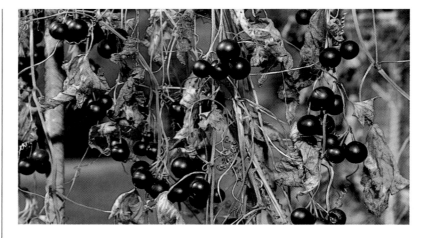

Aconite (Monk's hood)

Use for a dry cough that is accompanied by a high temperature and is triggered by a cold wind or by panic. The coughing begins suddenly, usually before midnight, with short, rough hacks. Inhaling produces a wheezing noise. Children are restless and very anxious. They hold onto their throats while coughing.

■ Dosage: 5 granules of *Aconite* 6C every hour in the beginning

Ipecacuanha (Root of ipecac)

Ipecacuanha helps, especially in warm, damp spring weather, but also after long exposure to cold winter air. A dry cough with breathing difficulties develops from a tickling irritation in the larynx; the white discharge can have a nasty taste that makes you sick. The cough can also be loose and coarsely rattling. The mucus is so tenacious that it is barely possible to cough it up. Food, bile, and blood can be vomited with the tongue remaining clean. The face can flush red or bluish, often accompanied by nosebleeds. Walking in cold air, warm rooms, and high temperatures worsens the condition. Cold drinks improve the condition.

■ Dosage: 5 granules of *Ipecacuanha* 6C every two hours

Good substances to use for chest compresses are lard, castor oil, and ricotta cheese.

Phosphorus (Phosphorus)

After colds accompanied by hoarseness or after overexertion, a burning, increasingly painful cough develops. Especially after getting up in the morning, the hoarseness can cause a complete loss of voice. The patient presses his hands against his chest. Lying down is only possible on the right side. If the patient turns onto his back or his left side in bed, a violent fit of coughing wakes him up. The patient craves cold or cold drinks for relief, but these only make the cough worse. Inhaling cold air, sudden changes in temperature, speaking, laughing, and crying make the condition worse. Lying on the right side relieves the symptoms.

■ Dosage: 5 granules of *Phosphorus* 6C three times a day

Drosera (Sundew)

The spasmodic and tickling cough can become so bad that it makes the patient vomit thick mucus. With the violent fits of coughing, the patient is barely able to breathe. He has a feeling of suffocation and a red, flushed face. The voice is remarkably deep and hoarse. Diarrhea occurs. The patient holds his chest in an effort to relieve the intolerable shooting pain. Children are often restless, anxious, and irritable. The symptoms are worse between midnight and 1 A.M. Speaking increases the irritation and leads to coughing.

■ Dosage: 5 granules of *Drosera* 6C three times a day

Spongia (Roasted sea sponge)

Spongia can help if the larynx is very sensitive to the touch and the voice is coarse and accompanied by a nervous cough with a compulsion to hawk. The dry, barking cough is incessant night and day, but the patient only coughs up a small amount of light mucus. There is a burning sensation in the chest. The patient is hungry and thirsty. At night, feelings of suffocation wake him up with a start. The condition is worse before and after midnight.

Excitement, cold drinks, lying down, and speaking or singing increase the symptoms. Sitting up in bed provides relief, as does eating and drinking, especially warm food and drink.

If you don't notice any improvement after taking three doses of a remedy, you should select the remedy which is most similar to the one you've been using or see your doctor or homeopath.

Consult an experienced homeopath in severe cases of chronic bronchial diseases or if the first two remedies you select do not help you.

Types of Coughs and Their Treatment

Type of Cough	Appropriate Remedy
Dry cough with high temperature and restlessness	Aconite
Colds affecting the bronchi	Phosphorus
Fits of spasmodic coughing with breathing difficulties and a red face	Drosera

---

■ Dosage: 5 granules of *Spongia* 6C every two hours

Chest Cough

A spasmodic cough appears without any other signs of a cold, although it can be a lingering symptom of a cold that was not treated with a suitable remedy.

■ Dosage: We recommend 3 granules of any of the following remedies three times a day in the potency 6C; after noticeable improvement, 5 granules once a day, fifteen minutes before breakfast, for a few more days

You can relieve a spasmodic cough that occurs while visiting the theatre, or going to a concert or similar event by chewing two or three juniper berries and then letting them melt in your mouth.

Bromium (Bromine)

Use *Bromium* to treat coughs, asthma, or diarrhea after warm days with cool evenings. The *Bromium* patient chills easily after sweating. Extreme hoarseness or even loss of voice is typical. Rattling breathing noises and a dry, spasmodic, wheezing cough appear. The inhaled air feels cold. The symptoms are worse when inhaling cold air and in warm rooms. They improve with cold drinks or at the seashore.

Conium (Poison hemlock)

You can use *Conium* to treat a persistent dry cough caused by a dry spot on the larynx. The coughing begins as soon as the patient reclines. The patient has to sit up at once and keeps coughing until the mucous has loosened, then the urge to cough disappears and sleep is possible. The slightest effort leads to difficulty in breathing. The symptoms are worse with speaking, laughing, and deep breathing. The cough also gets worse when the arms or hands become cold and when coming inside from the cold. Sitting up relieves the symptoms.

Sticta pulmonaria (Lungwort)

The cough is preceded by a cold. The mucous membranes of the nose are dry. There is a disagreeable feeling that the nose is blocked and a constant desire to blow the nose. The patient clears his throat to avoid coughing, but he cannot stop. The feeling of weariness is very marked. The symptoms are worse in the evening and at night. Lying down and deep breathing also increase the coughing.

Hyoscyamus (Henbane)

Hyoscyamus cures a dry, sometimes spasmodic cough that gets distinctly worse at night and usually begins immediately after lying down. Sensitive people often have this cough during times of

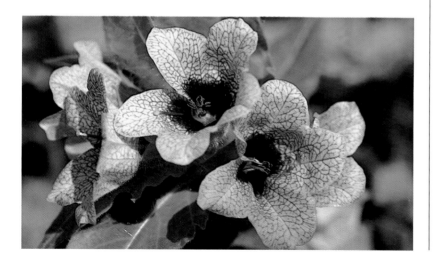

Hyoscyamus niger (Henbane) belongs to the nightshade family of plants. This homeopathic constitutional remedy is prepared from the whole plant while it is in bloom.

inner tension. Lying down or eating and drinking aggravates the condition. The symptoms improve in the daytime.

Diarrhea

When diarrhea is a symptom of another disease, be sure you drink a sufficient amount of liquids and have an appropriate diet. Avoid sweets, alcohol, and coffee, as well as fatty and spicy food. In severe or persistent cases of diarrhea, consult your doctor or practitioner.

Arsenicum album (Arsenic trioxide, White arsenic)
Arsenicum album relieves diarrhea caused by eating spoiled meat or fish, cold food, or ice cream. The stools are dark, foul smelling, and acrid. The patient feels terrible and very weak. At the same time he is restless, shaky, and anxious. He is often very thirsty, but he drinks only little sips. In some cases, the patient has a fainting spell before or after diarrhea. The condition is worse after eating or drinking and at night.

■ Dosage: 3 granules of *Arsenicum album* 12C every two hours

Pulsatilla (Wind flower)
Watery stools may occur with abdominal pains after fatty meals, after cold drinks with heavy meals, after fruit juice, or after overeating. Each of the stools is different. The patient is barely thirsty. Treat these cases with *Pulsatilla*.

■ Dosage: 5 granules of *Pulsatilla* 6C three times a day

Chamomilla (German chamomile)
Chamomilla is the best remedy if the diarrhea smells of rotten eggs and is greenish and slimy like chopped spinach or if the diarrhea occurs after stress, anger, or during teething. The patient is irritable, and nothing pleases him.

■ Dosage: 5 granules of *Chamomilla* 6C three times a day

In addition to the homeopathic treatment, you can eat grated apples or boiled and strained carrots. Another recipe that relieves diarrhea is blueberry tea. To prepare this, soak 2 tablespoons of dried and squashed blueberries in 1 pint (.5l) of cold water. Bring it to a boil and let it steep for ten minutes. Strain the tea and drink it in small portions all day.

Nux vomica (Poison nut)

Use *Nux vomica* to treat sickness and diarrhea that occur after overeating or eating indiscriminately, after too much alcohol, nicotine, or coffee, after misuse of laxatives, or after taking antibiotics. An important symptom is abdominal cramps with ineffectual urges to pass stool. The cramps feel better when the patient doubles over. The patient also often suffers from painful, itching hemorrhoids. The condition is worse in the morning and after meals. The patient feels better after expelling small amounts of stool, in the evenings, and when resting.

■ Dosage: 5 granules of *Nux vomica* three times a day

Veratrum album (White hellebore)

Veratrum album is an effective remedy for very painful diarrhea that occurs in the summer and fall with abundant stools that are either similar to rice water or are greenish and slimy. The stools can be mixed with blood and are odorless. The patient has cold sweats and a gaunt face. He feels cold, turns blue all over, and finally suffers a circulatory collapse with muscle cramps. He is extremely thirsty and drinks large amounts of cold water, which only aggravates the symptoms.

■ Dosage: 5 granules of *Veratrum album* 6C every two hours

Podophyllum (May apple)

Use *Podophyllum* to treat severe, painless diarrhea that occurs in the early morning, after eating sour fruit, during hot weather, and

Diarrhea draws a lot of fluid out of your body. Replace this by drinking noncarbonated mineral water. You should also take salt and sugar, about 1 teaspoon of each stirred into a glass of tea.

Diarrhea Is always Different

Diarrhea with	Appropriate Remedy
Weakness, anxiety	Arsenicum album
Nausea, cold sweats	Veratrum album
Nausea, heartburn, pains	Nux vomica
Watery discharges, spasms	Pulsatilla

during teething. The yellow or greenish, watery, foul-smelling stool is expelled explosively with flatulence. Before this occurs, there is a great deal of gurgling and rumbling in the stomach and abdomen. Afterwards, the patient is exhausted. The stomach is highly sensitive to the touch and to pressure from clothes. Sometimes, there is a peculiar link with headaches: either the headache and the diarrhea alternate, or there is headache in the summer and diarrhea in the winter. The condition is worse in the early morning, after eating or drinking (especially fruit or milk), in hot weather, or after taking a bath or washing. The patient feels better if he bends over or presses on the abdomen with the palm of his hand.

■ Dosage: 5 granules of *Podophyllum* 6C every two hours

Ipecacuanha (Root of ipecac)

Stools with a grass-green or scummy and fermented appearance can occur after eating indiscriminately, eating fatty meals, chewing tobacco, eating green fruit or ice cream in the summer and fall, and when hot days are followed by cold nights. *Ipecacuanha* can relieve persistent nausea and abdominal cramps with cutting pains in the navel area. The patient has a very pale face with dark rings under the eyes. The condition is worse after eating, drinking, or moving around.

■ Dosage: 5 granules of *Ipecacuanha* 6C every two hours

China (Peruvian bark)

China is recommended for painless diarrhea with a lot of flatulence that occurs in the summer after eating unripe fruit, drinking milk or beer, after giving birth, or during teething. *China* is also effective against chronic diarrhea in the elderly. The stool is watery with very little odor. Afterwards, the person is tired and drowsy. Continued weakness and a thirst for small amounts of drink are typical symptoms. The symptoms become worse after eating fruit. Using a hot-water bottle or doubling over alleviates some of the symptoms.

■ Dosage: 5 granules of *China* 6C three times a day

Warm or hot body compresses feel good and relieve diarrhea. Wrap a hot, damp cotton towel around your body from the chest down to the thighs. Then fold the ends together lightly over your stomach. Put a woolen blanket over this and cover yourself with your bedclothes. Leave the compress on for about an hour.

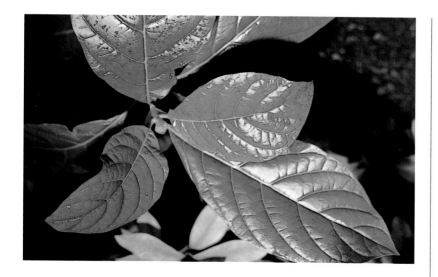

China *is prepared from Peruvian bark* (Cinchona succirubra *or* Cinchona pubescens). *It is used as a constitutional remedy for convalescence, anemia, chronic intestinal diseases, and diarrhea.*

Earache

Children frequently suffer from earaches; they usually occur at night and are very intense.

Aconite (Monk's hood)

Most cases of intense earache on the left side occur for a short period of time after ears are exposed to cold wind. Sometimes the pain begins shortly before midnight with a high fever. When the temperature begins to rise, shivering chills can occur. Afterwards, the skin is hot and dry, and the patient is restless and apprehensive.

■ Dosage: 3 granules of *Aconite* 6C every half hour; after improvement, increase the intervals

Aconitum compositum eardrops

The ear is red, hot, and extremely sensitive to noise. Children scream with pain; adults can bearly tolerate it. The condition gets worse at about 11 P.M. Being in a warm room increases the pain.

■ Dosage: 3 drops of the warmed fluid three times a day, in addition to *Aconite*

Press on the bony arch behind the ear to see if the pains have reached this region. If they have, you must consult a specialist. You must also call a doctor if the patient cannot raise his head when lying down or if raising his head is very painful. (The doctor may suspect meningitis.)

Pulsatilla (Wind flower)

Use *Pulsatilla* for earaches (usually on the right side) caused by cold or which follow a catarrh with an infection. The patient feels as if his ear is blocked. The external ear may be swollen and red. The patient is whiny, moody, and in need of loving care. The symptoms are worse in warm rooms, in the evening, and at night. They improve outdoors and in cool places.

■ Dosage: 3 granules of *Pulsatilla* 6C every two hours

Apis mellifica (Honeybee)

Use *Apis* to treat burning, stinging pains that occur when swallowing. These are often accompanied by a sore throat. Typically, there is a pink swelling of the eardrum, and the effusion in the middle ear shows through. The throat and uvula may also be swollen. The symptoms are worse with warmth, with touch, on swallowing, and with chewing. They improve with cold and with cold applications to the ear.

■ Dosage: 3 granules of *Apis mellifica* 6C every half hour

Belladonna (Deadly nightshade)

Belladonna is the remedy for intense, throbbing pains, predominantly on the right side. The patient's ear or head is red, and the pupils are dilated. There is a feeling of heat and fullness in the ear and face. Children suddenly begin to cry while playing. The throbbing, hammering, or pulsating pain subsides after a few minutes. The patient feels as if he is "burning up" but stays covered in bed. The symptoms are worse with cold, light, and vibration. They improve with warmth.

■ Dosage: 3 granules of *Belladonna* 6C every half hour

Chamomilla (German chamomile)

We use this remedy primarily for teething infants. The symptoms are one red cheek and one pale one. Some children also complain of a sore throat. The patient always wants to be carried around and is restless and ill-tempered. The symptoms are worse before mid-

You can relieve an earache by putting a small bag filled with a chopped medium-sized onion on the ear. When cold applications are not recommended, you can enhance the effect of the onion by heating the onion in a dry frying pan and cooling it down to body temperature.

night, with warmth, with warm drinks, and when stooping. The pains are relieved if you caress the child and carry him around. Motion also improves the condition.

▪ Dosage: 3 granules of *Chamomilla* 6C every half hour

Ferrum phosphoricum (Ferrum phosphate)

Use *Ferrum phosphoricum* with a drawing earache in the early stage of an inflammation. Also use it if the middle ear is red, hot, swollen, and painful. The temperature rises slowly up to a maximum of 102°F (39°C). The symptoms are worse at night, especially from 4 to 6 A.M. They improve with cold applications and with walking around slowly.

▪ Dosage: 3 granules of *Ferrum phosphoricum* 12C every hour

Gelsemium (Yellow jasmine)

Gelsemium relieves a sharp or shooting earache that comes and goes. It often appears as an aftermath of a cold and is usually on the right side. The patient also complain of shooting pains in the throat that extend to the ear when swallowing. The symptoms are aggravated when sitting.

▪ Dosage: 5 granules of *Gelsemium* 6C every two hours

Eczema

In treating eczema and eruptions of the skin, many remedies are worth considering. We have confined ourselves to the most important ones. If you cannot find the remedy you've been using listed here, please seek advice from an experienced homeopath.

Sulphur (Sulphur)

Sulphur helps with eczema and psoriasis. The dry, scaly, reddened or dirty-looking patches on the skin alternately burn and itch. The patient scratches until the affected areas bleed. The patient often uses cortisone ointments to relieve the condition. However, when the treatement is stopped, the eruptions break out again very

Your pharmacist and your homeopath will be glad to help you select the correct remedies for a homeopathic first-aid kit especially suited to your requirements.

If eruptions of the skin disappear after using preparations containing cortisone, new and different skin complaints can ensue, for example, greasy skin, dandruff, cracks, or diseases of other organs.

Hepar sulphuris (Calcium sulphide) is effective against moist rashes in the folds of skin and in the bends of joints. These are susceptible to cracks and festering. They bleed easily and are sensitive to cold and to touch. Foul-smelling pus and wounds that heal poorly are also characteristic. Dosage: 3 granules of *Hepar sulphuris* 12C twice a day.

quickly. The condition is worse in the warmth of a bed or after contact with water. Scratching affects the skin adversely. The symptoms improve in fresh air.

■ Dosage: 5 granules of *Sulphur* 6C twice a day

Rhus toxicodendron (Poison ivy)

Rhus toxicodendron is suitable for treating contact eczema from metals, synthetic fibers, and rubber, as well as hives, cold sores on the lips, shingles, and chickenpox. The symptoms are worse in damp cold weather, cold drafts, and cold water. The condition improves in hot water.

■ Dosage: 5 granules of *Rhus toxicodendron* 6C twice a day

Graphites (Graphite)

Graphites helps with damp, sticky rashes that occur in the bends of joints and behind the ears. These discharge a honeylike fluid. The itching is aggravated by warmth. *Graphites* is also effective against painful cracks on the fingers, the anus, the nipples, in the corners of the mouth and the eyes, between the toes, and in injuries that tend to fester.

■ Dosage: 3 granules of *Graphites* 12C twice a day

Fainting

Fainting occurs when the blood supply to the brain does not provide enough oxygen. The patient falls down, assuming a position which ensures more oxygen gets to the brain. You should move the patient into the fresh air, lay him down on his back, and loosen or open any tight clothing.

■ Dosage: Apply the indicated remedies in a dilution of 30C (dissolve 3 granules in a little water), dip in a handkerchief, and hold under the unconscious person's nose. Also dab on the cheeks and forehead and wet the lips. If possible, put 3 granules on the tongue.

Aconite (Monk's hood)

Use *Aconite* when something happens suddenly, such as fainting, collapse, shock, sudden fright, bad news, or unexpected excitement.

Coffea (Coffee)

Coffea revives the patient who has fainted after hearing good news. Before fainting, the person perceives everything with a heightened awareness; he laughs and cries with joy or emotion.

Pulsatilla (Wind flower)

Use *Pulsatilla* to treat fainting that occurs in warm, poorly aired, or overcrowded rooms. *Pulsatilla* is also helpful for women who faint during menstruation, especially after they have been standing for a long time.

Nux vomica (Poison nut)

This is effective for fainting due to excessive straining with painful stools, continued overexertion, stress, lack of sleep, or strong smells.

If the fainting fit continues for longer than a few minutes, the patient must be treated by a doctor immediately.

Give *Chamomilla* (German chamomile) if a person faints from anger or from intense pain.

Nux moschata (Nutmeg) is often helpful if the sight of blood makes you faint.

Fever

Fever can occur with many illnesses. Thus, you should wait a while and observe the symptoms of the disease. If the fever continues and you can definitely assign the symptoms to a remedy, use the remedy in the appropriate way. If you are not sure, consult an experienced homeopath. You can find additional advice under the headings "Catarrh," "Cold," "Cough," "Earache," and "Sore Throat."

Belladonna (Deadly nightshade)

Use *Belladonna* if the fever develops suddenly and begins with a loss of appetite and fatigue. When the patient wakes up, the first symptoms are a fiery red, glowing face with dilated pupils, throbbing headache, perspiration, a sensation of being very hot in bed,

If the temperature is over 103° F (39.5° C), if the pain increases drastically, or if the general condition deteriorates, you should always consult your doctor or homeopath.

In an *Aconite* condition, the fever should go down, and the patient should calm down in half an hour to an hour.

If you are no better after three or four doses, select another remedy or consult your practioner.

and an immediate chill when the blankets are removed. The patient wants to stay covered up. His hands and feet seem cold. The mucous membranes are bright red and later become dark red and blotchy. The arteries in the throat and temples pulsate visibly. The patient is tormented by nightmares from which he awakes abruptly.

■ Dosage: 3 granules of *Belladonna* 6C every half hour

Aconitum (Monk's hood)

After exposure to cold wind, sudden anxiety, or a shocking experience, a violent onset of fever of 104° F (40° C) or more can occur. If the patient has gone to bed without symptoms, the fever usually begins with shivering chills shortly before midnight. Because the patient is anxious and restless, he can only sleep for short spells. His face is red when lying down, but it becomes pale when he sits up.

■ Dosage: 3 granules of *Aconitum* 6C every half hour

Ferrum phosphoricum (Ferrum phosphate)

The fever rises slowly to a temperature of about 102° F (39° C). The patient usually has no catarrh or chill and has no serious impairment to his general state of health. After sleeping, his complexion is red; otherwise it keeps changing, especially when he changes position. The condition is often accompanied by nosebleeds.

■ Dosage: 3 granules of *Ferrum phosphoricum* 12C every hour

Measures to Reduce Fever

■ Place compresses around the legs and chest; wash the upper part of the body, but make sure that the parts in question remain warm.

■ Give an enema with about 16 ounces (500ml) of water or chamomile tea. The temperature of the liquid should be about 1° below body temperature.

Flatulence

Eating too quickly, eating flatulent foods (such as beans, peas, some sorts of cabbage, and unusual foods), or swallowing air can lead to the development of gas in the gastrointestinal tract. This is often very painful. Flatulence is usually accompanied by loud intestinal rumbling. In addition, a full feeling in the stomach, general pain in the abdomen, and irregular stools can accompany it.

Lycopodium (Club moss)

Flatulence begins during the meal or shortly afterwards, especially after consuming milk, sweets, pastries, onions, and garlic. In addition, there is a clearly audible bubbling, fermenting, or rumbling, especially in the lower abdomen. The gas is usually odorless and is passed easily when moving. Burping does not relieve the complaints. Belts or other tight garments around the waist aggravate the symptoms.

■ Dosage: 5 granules of *Lycopodium* 6C twice a day

Carbo vegetabilis (Vegetable charcoal)

Use *Carbo vegetabilis* for flatulence with a foul odor and pains in the whole abdomen with burping. The patient has a burning stomachache that radiates to the spine between the shoulder blades. He feels full after a few bites of food. Digestion is incomplete, and the symptoms are worse when the patient moves or sits in an upright position. Burping provides relief.

■ Dosage: 3 granules of *Carbo vegetabilis* 12C twice a day

China (Peruvian bark)

A treatment with *China* can help when flatulence is caused by eating gassy food or drinking milk. Passing gas provides no relief. Another indication is a sour or bitter burping. The patient has a feeling of fullness after a few bites of food or feels as if the food were stuck in the throat. Diarrhea with undigested stools and intense flatulence occur, especially after eating fruit and sour foods. The symptoms are worse after meals that include milk and juicy fruit. Touching the stomach and the abdomen makes the condition worse. Applying warmth or doubling up improves the symptoms.

■ Dosage: 5 granules of *China* 6C twice a day

Nux vomica (Poison nut)

Nux vomica is effective for flatulence accompanied by constipation or diarrhea and violent spasms after overeating, drinking alcohol or coffee, from stressful situations, or from lack of exercise. The patient has the feeling that a stone is pressing on his stomach. This feeling persists for three hours after eating. The symptoms get worse after heavy or large meals. Doubling up and passing small amounts of stool provide relief.

■ Dosage: 5 granules of *Nux vomica* 6C twice a day

Flu-like Symptoms

You can usually treat flu-like symptoms quite well at home with the following remedies. You can accelerate the process of recovery with light meals, preferably a diet that includes plenty of fruit juice. The treatment of influenza is best left to a doctor or homeopath. After your temperature has returned to normal, you should stay at home for another day. Refer to "Catarrh," "Colds," "Cough," and "Fever" for further information.

Rhus toxicodendron (Poison ivy)

The symptoms develop as a result of overexertion and of getting very wet or cold in damp, cold weather. The patient has severe pains in the muscles and joints and feels extremely weak. He wants to lie down but is very restless due to the rheumatic pains. Stiffness can develop in the early morning, while resting, and when cooling down. Nettle rash or herpes often ensues.

■ Dosage: 5 granules of *Rhus toxicodendron* 6C three times a day

If flatulence continues and becomes chronic, a yeast fungi (such as *Candida albicans*) may be affecting the intestinal tract. To ascertain this, the doctor or homeopath has to do a special stool examination to be able to take the appropriate measures.

After a feverish disease, you should stay at home for a full day after the temperature has gone down to 98.6° F (37° C), or you could suffer a relapse.

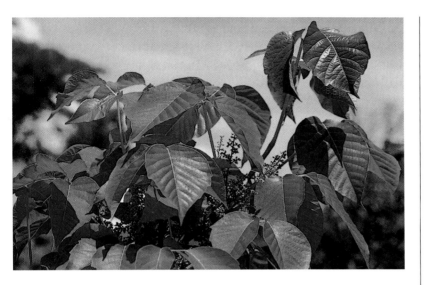

Rhus toxicodendron is the Latin term for poison ivy. This plant is actually poisonous. Thus, it is used almost exclusively in homeopathy, where it loses its danger because it is very diluted.

Gelsemium (Yellow jasmine)

In the spring or in warm weather, flu-like symptoms usually develop as a result of exposure to cold. The patient's temperature rises slowly. After one or two days, severe pains in the head, back, and limbs set in. Shivering fits run along the spine, and the teeth chatter. Additional symptoms include a red, swollen face, dizziness, a sore throat, a feeling of heaviness, and weariness. The patient is sensitive to light and doesn't want to move around.

■ Dosage: 5 granules of *Gelsemium* 6C three times a day

Eupatorium perfoliatum (Thoroughwort)

The patient's whole body aches, and he feels exhausted. The legs and head in particular are very painful. The joints feel as if they were sprained. Coughing is so painful that the patient holds his chest. The face is red and hot. Pains in the right area of the stomach can also occur. Before feeling chilled, the patient is very thirsty for cold drinks. After the chill, the patient often vomits.

■ Dosage: 5 granules of *Eupatorium perfoliatum* 6C three times a day

With all kinds of colds, it is important to drink a great deal. Ideally, you should drink fruit juices mixed with water, fruit and herb teas, and mildly diuretic tea.

Gallbladder Problems

Fatty meals, eating hastily, and prolonged anger or stress disturb the formation and flow of bile. At first, the stool is too soft and too light in color. This is followed by a feeling of increasing pressure under the ribs on the right.

Atropinum sulphuricum (Atropine sulphate)

Atropinum sulphuricum has an antispasmodic effect if there is a feeling of pressure, a stitch, or spasmodic pains on the right side of the abdomen.

- ■ Dosage: 3 granules of *Atropinum sulphuricum* 4C every fifteen minutes

Magnesium phosphoricum (Magnesium phosphate)

Magnesium phosphoricum is effective against gallstone pain with severe flatulence that forces the patient to double over. Burping does not relieve the pain. Because of his bloated abdomen, he has to loosen his clothing. The patient improves with warmth, rubbing, or pressing. Passing gas while walking also provides relief.

- ■ Dosage: 3 granules of *Magnesium phosphoricum* 12C every hour

Colocynthis (Bitter cucumber)

Spasmodic pains in the stomach extend to the lower back or the pubic region. These are triggered by anger or insult but also by cold drinks, physical overexertion, and overheating. Cold and stretching aggravate the condition. Pulling the legs up or doubling over provides relief. Pressure or a hot-water bottle on the affected area also helps relieve the cramps.

- ■ Dosage: 5 granules of *Colocynthis* 6C every hour

Pulsatilla (Wind flower)

Gallstone attacks that occur after eating very fatty foods or after warm meals with cold drinks respond very well to *Pulsatilla*. Fre-

---

In addition to taking the appropriate remedy, the factors that cause the illness should be changed.

If you have problems with your gallbladder, you should avoid the following foods: animal fats (including butter), fried food, egg yolks, and ice-cold drinks.

quently, there is a bitter, putrid, or rancid burping and vomiting. The symptoms improve with fresh air and exercise.

■ Dosage: 5 granules of *Pulsatilla* 6C every hour

Chelidonium (Greater celandine)

Use *Chelidonium* for gallbladder problems accompanied by a bloated abdomen and a feeling that the abdomen is constricted with a string. This kind of gallbladder problem is often preceded by a backache in the area of the right shoulder blade or by stiffness and tension in the neck, usually on the left side. Hot drinks and warm milk alleviate the condition. Eating also makes the patient feel better for a short period of time.

■ Dosage: 5 granules of *Chelidonium* 6C three times a day

Bleeding Gums

If the slightest touch of the toothbrush leads to bleeding gums or if taking a bite of a crunchy apple has the same effect, then you should remember Samuel Hahnemann's useful pellets. In addition, don't be afraid to visit your dentist. He is the only person who can tell whether you're gums are infected.

Arnica (Leopard's bane)

You can cure frequent bleeding with *Arnica*.

■ Dosage: 3 granules of *Arnica* 6C two to three times a day

Nux vomica (Poison nut)

Use *Nux vomica* when the gums are swollen and whitish. The teeth ache with cold food or drinks, when chewing, in cold air, and when air is drawn through the teeth. You can also use *Nux vomica* for canker sores with bloody saliva. The patient is very tense at work and at home. He appears irritable and is very sensitive to noises, smells, light, and other disturbances.

■ Dosage: 5 granules of *Nux vomica* 6C twice a day

Bleeding gums may indicate that you should have any amalgam fillings replaced. They may also be a symptom that your mouth and intestines are infested with fungi. In any case, you should have your mouth examined.

Nux moscata (Nutmeg) cures headaches and an extremely bloated stomach with flatulence caused by overeating. Fainting can occur during or after passing stool. The patient can sleep in any position because he is so drowsy.

Hangover, Overeating

After an excessive intake of alcoholic drinks or overeating (often combined with smoky air), you feel deathly ill the next day. The following remedies can offer relief.

■ Dosage: 3 granules 6C of the indicated remedy every hour until you feel some relief

Nux vomica (Poison nut)

Nux vomica is known as the Alka-Seltzer of homeopathy. If you experience heartburn and headache after excessive alcohol, tobacco, or coffee, or if you have heartburn after overeating or eating too hastily, *Nux vomica* is often helpful. The patient is agitated or angry. Often he vomits. The stomach region is very sensitive to pressure. The patient usually uses a large amount of antacids. The symptoms are worse in the morning and one or two hours after eating. They are better in the evening and with rest.

Pulsatilla (Wind flower)

Nausea and spasmodic abdominal pains and headache occur after overeating, after eating heavy and fatty meals, after eating pork or ice cream, and after drinking ice cold drinks. Typically, there is no thirst. The symptoms are worse in warm, closed rooms and are relieved by fresh air and exercise.

Heartburn

The wine is too dry, the meal is too fatty, and the meeting is too hectic. These are just a few of the many reasons for painful and troublesome heartburn.

■ Dosage: 3 granules 6C of the following remedies whenever you feel the need (use 12C for *Carbo vegetabilis* and *Magnesium phosphoricum*)

Robinia (Locust)

The main remedy for heartburn is *Robinia*. It is especially useful in cases where the heartburn is so bad that burping produces sour gastric juices which dull the teeth. It is also effective in cases of intolerance to fat that become worse at night. Clay with healing properties is a good household remedy for heartburn. It absorbs excess gastric juices, bile, toxic substances, and intestinal bacteria.

Iris versicolor (Blue flag)

Heartburn that is accompanied by profuse saliva responds well to *Iris versicolor*. The effect also extends to the stomach, intestines, pancreas, and saliva glands. The heartburn may be accompanied by a migraine headache.

Calcium carbonicum (Calcium carbonate) helps with heartburn that produces a sour taste in the mouth.

Nux vomica (Poison nut)

Nux vomica is the appropriate remedy for a feeling of fullness that occurs after meals. Usually the patient feels nauseous and has a sour, bitter taste in his mouth. *Nux vomica* is especially suited to overachievers.

Lycopodium (Club moss)

If heartburn occurs after small meals and is often accompanied by

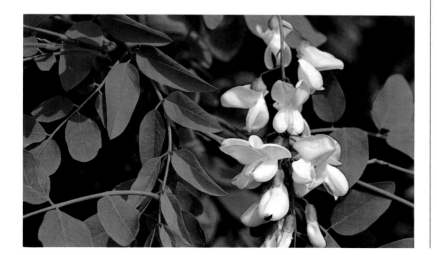

The locust tree (Robinia pseudoacacia) *is also known as false acacia. It belongs to the pea family and has white, fragrant blossoms rich in nectar. The locust tree is the source of the remedy* Robinia.

Heartburn with hiccups,
retching, and a thirst for
cold drinks indicates the
use of *Magnesium
phosphoricum*.

spasmodic pain, use *Lycopodium*. Characteristically, the heartburn appears from 4 to 8 P.M.

Acidum carbolicum (Carbolic acid)

Acidum carbolicum may help if the stomach is bloated and a disagreeable hot flush rises up the esophagus. Typically, the patient craves coffee and tobacco.

Carbo vegetabilis (Vegetable charcoal)

Use this remedy when the heartburn is accompanied by violent flatulence. The patient chills easily, his lips are bluish, and he feels better in the fresh air.

Hemorrhoids

Hemorrhoids occur when the circulation in the portal vein becomes restricted. This often points to a malfunction in the digestive system, especially in the metabolism of the liver.

Aesculus (Horse chestnut)

Try *Aesculus* if you have external or internal hemorrhoids that barely bleed and that are accompanied by burning or shooting pains in the rectum and itching at night. Usually a sensation of congestion in the sacral region follows with severe pains. These are worse after passing stool, taking long walks, and standing. During pregnancy and menstruation, the condition becomes worse. The condition improves in warm weather.

■ Dosage: 7 granules of *Aesculus* 4C three times a day

With hemorrhoids you
should eat only light meals
in the evening and drink
one or two cups of a liver-
and-bile tea.

Nux vomica (Poison nut)

Use *Nux vomica* to treat internal hemorrhoids that itch badly and rarely bleed. A sedentary lifestyle, overindulging in coffee, tobacco, alcohol, and similar substances, and abusing drugs (for example, laxatives) lead to constipation with frequent ineffective urges to pass stool. Often the patient has lower back pain. The condition

What Helps Relieve Hemorrhoids

■ Washing the anal region with cold water in the shower relieves the itching.

■ Sitz baths with oak bark have an astringent and anti-inflammatory effect.

■ Make sure your digestion is regular and your stool is soft; eat large amounts of linseed or bran.

■ Avoid warm and heavy meals after 6 P.M.

is worse with touching, after passing stool, after walking, with excitement, and after drinking beer. The condition improves with short, cold applications.

■ Dosage: 5 granules of *Nux vomica* 6C twice a day

Hamamelis (Witch hazel)

The large external hemorrhoids feel sore and rough. They pulsate and are very sensitive to the touch. Often dark red coagulated blood appears. After the hemorrhage, the patient feels weak and has headaches and a backache. He feels as if his back were breaking.

■ Dosage: 7 granules of *Hamamelis* 4C three times a day

Paeonia (Peony)

Inflamed hemorrhoids with fissures, painful ulcers, or fistulae and an oozing secretion are very sensitive to the touch. They cause intense pain in the anal region during and after emptying the bowels and when walking. Because of the pain, the patient often suppresses the urge to pass stool, and this leads to constipation.

■ Dosage: 7 granules of *Paenoia* 4C three times a day

Remedies containing *Hamamelis* are especially suited for the external treatment of hemorrhoids, as for instance *Hamamelis* ointment or suppositories. They can be purchased at any pharmacy.

Hoarseness

Hoarseness is often the main feature of a cold in the larynx area or of overexerting the voice, but it can also be a symptom of a bad cold.

■ Dosage: We recommend 3 granules of the indicated remedy in the 6th potency three times a day. If no improvement is evident, consult your homeopath.

Chamomilla (German chamomile)

The symptoms are stiff mucus in the throat, dryness, burning, and thirst. A tickling in the throat starts a cough. The temperature rises in the evening. The patient is restless or in a discontented mood and does not want to speak.

Nux vomica (Poison nut)

Use *Nux vomica* for hoarseness, tension, and pain in the throat. Dryness in the throat leads to a rough, dry, and deep cough that does not produce mucus. The patient has a sullen and quarrelsome disposition and is stubborn and headstrong.

Pulsatilla (Wind flower)

Typical symptoms are a sore throat and a feeling of soreness in the

Phytolacca americana (Pokeweed) is very effective for inflammations of the throat and inflammations of the sciatic nerve.

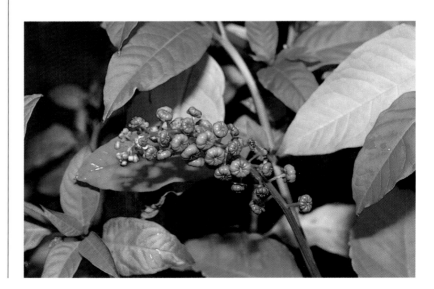

roof of the mouth. The patient may have catarrh with profuse yellow, green, or yellow green, smelly discharge. He has bad breath in the morning and a loose cough (which may be dry at night) with pain in the chest. The patient feels better in fresh, cold air, and his condition improves. Desires and complaints vary greatly.

Capsicum (Cayenne pepper)
Use when hoarseness is accompanied by a tickling in the nose and a stuffy nose or by a cough with occasional pain.

Apis mellifica (Honeybee)
Due to hoarseness, the larynx is very sensitive. The rough, dry sensation in the throat improves with cold drinks. Exercise makes the patient short of breath.

Sambucus (Elder)
Treat hoarseness accompanied by deep, hollow coughing that produces no mucus with *Sambucus*. Frequent yawning, restlessness, and thirst are also characteristic.

Carbo vegetabilis (Vegetable charcoal)
Prolonged hoarseness that is worse in the mornings or evenings, after long or loud talking, or is a side effect of measles, responds well to *Carbo vegetabilis*.
◼ Dosage: 3 granules of *Carbo vegetabilis* 12C twice a day

Causticum (Potassium hydrate)
Use *Causticum* when hoarseness lasts so long that the patient has recovered from almost all of his other symptoms. It is also effective in cases of cough and cold where the whole chest is sore and painful. Sometimes the throat is also sore.

Silicea (Quartz)
Silicea is useful in cases where hoarseness and a prolonged catarrh occur because the patient's feet are cold.

Mercurius solubilis (Mercury) helps if the patient is tormented by a burning and tickling in the larynx. This is accompanied by disagreeable spells of sweating, especially at night. Breathing cold air worsens the condition.

Treat a rough sensation in the throat and a sore throat that is worse in the morning and improves as you speak with *Rhus toxicodendron* (Poison ivy). Additional symptoms are frequent sneezing, profuse mucus but no actual catarrh, and a shortness of breath.

Insect Bites and Stings

Mosquitoes seem to be unerringly attracted to certain people. Perhaps they have "sweet blood."

■ Dosage: 3 granules of the indicated remedy (except *Staphisagria*) in the potency 6C every half hour; after improvement, 3 granules every two to three hours

Apis mellifica (Honeybee)

If the sting causes symptoms similar to those of a bee sting, *Apis* will relieve the pink, watery, hot swelling and the stinging pain. The symptoms are worse in the sun, with warmth, and in a warm bed. You can relieve them with cold compresses.

Ledum (Marsh tea)

Ledum is especially appropriate after mosquito or horsefly bites that itch, burn, and swell. It is also effective when insect bites become septic. The puncture is cold to the touch, or the patient feels as if it were cold. The symptoms are worse with warmth and are relieved with cold applications.

Caladium (American arum)

Treat insect bites that itch and burn intensely with *Caladium*. The sweetish odor of sweat attracts insects.

Hypericum (St. John's wort)

Hypericum combats the intense pain of a puncture wound. You can also use *Hypericum* when the patient experiences a feeling of numbness and a general feeling of aggravation from cold.

Staphisagria (Stavesacre)

This homeopathic first-aid remedy has also proved useful against insect bites.

■ Dosage: 5 granules of *Staphisagria* 3C three times a day

In addition to *Apis* (Honeybee), you can dab an insect bite with a mother tincture of *Arnica* (Leopard's bane) or *Calendula* (Marigold). You can also use Dr. Bach's Rescue Remedy or tea tree oil. These remedies provide quick relief.

Insomnia

After a period of time, people who suffer from sleeplessness and who have to resort to strong drugs begin to dread the night hours. The dose of sleeping pills usually has to be increased. In such a case, it is essential that you consult your doctor or homeopath. Always bear in mind that the amount of sleep needed varies significantly from one person to another. If you only suffer from insomnia now and then, you can take the remedies listed here in the indicated dosage.

■ Dosage: 3 granules 6C of the indicated remedy once half an hour before going to bed (can be repeated if required)

Kali phosphoricum (Postassium phosphate)

Use *Kali phosphoricum* in cases where insomnia occurs after a long period of excitement, overwork, or worry and is accompanied by a feeling that even minor tasks are too much. This remedy prevents nightmares and sleepwalking.

Chamomilla (German chamomile)

Chamomilla is particularly effective in calming whiny children who always want to be carried around.

Coffea (Coffee)

Use *Coffea* if the patient cannot sleep because of intense joy or because he is excited about a future pleasurable event. His mind is filled with thoughts, and he cannot unwind. *Coffea* works well in these cases.

Ignatia (St. Ignatious bean)

If you are tormented by grief, disappointment, or shock, take *Ignatia*. Indications for using this remedy are frequent sighing, sobbing, moaning, and irritability with paradoxical reactions. The mental and physical condition can easily be reversed.

Persistent insomnia often masks depression or an organic illness.

Serious cases of sleeplessness in children often
reflect a traumatic birth
experience.

Nux vomica (Poison nut)

Nux vomica works especially well with the kind of sleeplessness that occurs after overwork and stress. *Nux vomica* is also suitable for irritable people who are often angry. It calms down patients who have indulged in too much coffee, nicotine, or alcohol.

Lumbago

Prolonged emotional tension with corresponding tenseness in the back, the effects of cold, or an awkward movement can lead to severe pains in the back.

■ Dosage: 5 granules of the indicated remedy in the 6th potency three times a day

Lumbago often indicates a
prolonged emotional
strain. If you have had to
deal with a great deal of
stress, overwork, problems
at work, problems with
your partner, worry, or
grief, you should counter
this strain with relaxation
exercises. Try biofeedback,
yoga, and progressive
muscle relaxation using
the Jacobson and
Feldenkrais methods.

Arnica (Leopard's bane)

Arnica is the first remedy for lumbago if the back feels sore, contorted, or exhausted after overexertion. The pain seems to spread all over the body, and the patient wants to be left alone. Movement and touch increase the severity of the symptoms. Lying flat relieves the pain.

Rhus toxicodendron (Poison ivy)

The lower back aches and feels torn or contorted. The symptoms appear after overexertion (for example, carrying heavy loads) or getting cold or wet. The symptoms are worse in bed in the mornings, from the effects of cold, and at the onset of every movement. Continued movement or applying warmth and massages relieves the pain.

Nux vomica (Poison nut)

After working in a stooped position in a draft, the lumbar portion of the spine aches, and the patient can only walk when bending forward. To turn over in bed, he first has to sit up. The patient is irritable, oversensitive, and easily loses his temper. The symptoms are worse at night and in the morning. The pains are aggravated by touch, cold, straining to pass stool, stooping, or straightening. Warmth and absolute rest improve the symptoms.

Bryonia (Wild hops, White bryony)
A twisting movement triggers the pain. This occurs after getting chilled while being overheated. The patient has severe pain when moving and is extremely irritable. The smallest movement increases the pain. Pressure (for example, lying on the painful spot) and cold provide relief.

Nervous Disorders

If nervousness is due to illness, you can use one of the following remedies as an additional measure if the description fits your condition.

■ Dosage: 5 granules 6C of the indicated remedy two to three times a day

Kali phosphoricum (Potassium phosphate)
Use *Kali phosphoricum* to treat nervous and physical exhaustion with a poor memory, despondency, and irritability. It is also effective if the smallest task becomes a major problem. The patient complains of headaches with dizziness and poor vision after a great mental effort. The symptoms are worse in the mornings, with any agitation, or with exertion. They improve with rest, warmth, and after meals.

Zincum valerianium (Valerinate of zinc)
Zincum valerianium calms nervous people who are suffering from depression due to exhaustion and who cannot keep still. If restlessness in the legs occurs at night, it disturbs the patient's sleep. The smallest amount of wine worsens the general state of well-being and the other symptoms.

Additional measures to reduce nervousness include alternating hot and cold showers, exercising in the fresh air, eating nutritious food, replacing fillings containing amalgam, and reducing electromagnetic radiation by turning off the television set or computer as often as possible.

Additional Homeopathic Remedies for Nervous Disorders

Acidum phosphoricum
Use in cases of nervous weakness after mental or physical overexertion, with prolonged grief, with acute diseases, in periods of rapid growth, and in conditions of indifference, apathy, poor concentration, or poor memory.

Kali bromatum (Potassium bromide)
Use in cases of nervous restlessness with failing memory and nightmares combined with a constant urge to move the hands and in cases when the symptoms are worse with mental effort but improve with physical exercise.

Valeriana (Valerian root)
Nervousness with extreme mood changes responds to *Valeriana*. Additional symptoms are irritability and sleeplessness. *Valeriana* also helps if sickness and diarrhea occur after anger.

Neuralgia

Persistent neuralgic pains can be exhausting. The particular homeopathic remedy that matches the patient and his symptoms can often offer very quick relief.

Aconitum napellus (Monk's hood)
After exposure to dry cold, anxious people can suddenly experience intense neuralgia, often in the region of the trigeminal (facial) nerve, with prickling and numbness.
■ Dosage: 3 granules of *Aconitum napellus* 6C every half hour

Magnesium phosphoricum (Magnesium phosphate)
Magnesium phosphoricum relieves pain that occurs in spasms, usu-

ally affecting the face, teeth, ears, or sciatic nerve. The pain bores its way along the course of the nerve. The condition becomes worse at night, with cold, cold bathing, swimming, soft touch, and draft. The symptoms improve with warmth, warm baths, warm compresses, and pressure.

■ Dosage: 5 granules of *Magnesium phosphoricum* 12C every hour

Hypericum (St. John's-wort)

Hypericum alleviates neuralgic pains after serious cuts and amputations. It is also good for squashed fingertips if you've applied *Arnica* (Leopard's bane) beforehand. You can also use *Hypericum* for neuralgia of the nerve root caused by diseases of the spine and the spinal cord, for pains in the coccyx after giving birth, for numbness, and for tingling sensations. The symptoms are worse at night, in the early morning, and in dampness and fog. They improve with rubbing and rest.

■ Dosage: 5 granules of *Hypericum* 6C two to three times a day

Mezereum (Spurge olive)

This is the remedy for burning, sharp, shooting, or twitching pains followed by numbness. These complaints arise after skin eruptions have subsided, especially if the skin eruptions have been suppressed by ointments. The symptoms are worse at night, in damp and cold weather, after washing with cold water, with changes of weather, and with touch. The symptoms improve if the patient is wrapped up and kept warm.

■ Dosage: 5 granules of *Mezereum* 6C twice a day

Overweight

You can carefully work out a diet to lose weight, but diets always have one big disadvantage: As soon you end the diet, you usually put on the pounds that you worked so hard to loose. If you just want to eat a little less for a while, you can support your good intentions with the following homeopathic remedies.

■ Dosage: 3 granules 6C (12C for *Calcium carbonicum* and *Graphites*) of the indicated remedy three times a day

Ammonium carbonicum (Ammonium carbonate)
Ammonium carbonicum helps the overweight patient who often feels tired. This patient catches cold easily, suffers from a weak heart, and experiences a feeling of heaviness in all his organs. He has a huge appetite but is satisfied after a few mouthfuls. Severe flatulence with intestinal rumbling is also characteristic.

Calcium carbonicum (Calcium carbonate)
The patient puts on a little weight especially from milk and milk products. There is a tendency to be constipated. Overwork leads to a loss of appetite or ravenous hunger. The patient often suffers from sour burping, colds when the weather changes, sour smelling sweat on the body and feet with the slightest exertion, and sweating at night, especially on the head.

Graphites (Graphite)
Graphites may help when the patient is overweight as a result of constant eating and a lack of exercise is accompanied by constipation. He has a burning stomachache that is only temporarily relieved by food or hot milk. Various skin eruptions can occur, often discharging a sticky, honeylike fluid. Fissures and cracks in the skin are also typical symptoms.

Capsicum (Cayenne pepper)
Capsicum is suitable for the overweight person who has flabby skin and tissues. He is lethargic, dislikes physical exercise, wants to do only routine tasks, and is easily homesick. He has a tendency to be unclean.

If you are worried about your surplus pounds, you should analyze your eating habits. Do without candy and reduce your intake of alcohol. If you are a beer drinker, switch to a light or alcohol-free beer. Substitute fresh fruit and vegetables for sweets.

Restlessness

Combating nervousness and restlessness is difficult even with homeopathy. Try to do without sedatives. If the remedies listed here do not produce the desired effect, please speak with your homeopathic doctor or practitioner. Remember that you can achieve relaxation through self-hypnosis.

■ Dosage: If required, take 5 granules twice a day in the potency 6C (12C for *Arsenicum album* and *Zincum metallicum*)

Arsenicum album (Arsenic trioxide, White arsenic)

Arsenicum album is useful when restlessness is combined with weakness and exhaustion after the slightest exertion. The patient is extremely apprehensive and is often easily chilled.

Kali bromatum (Potassium bromide)

Kali bromatum calms the urge to move and helps if mental efforts make the patient even more restless. It has proved to be a successful deterrent for nightmares. The patient's memory appears to be failing, and the patient gradually calms down only after physical exercise.

Aconite (Monk's hood)

Aconite is an effective remedy for restlessness combined with a high fever and a fear of dying.

Zincum metallicum (Metallic zinc)

Zincum metallicum can help in cases where the patient moves his legs incessantly in bed at night. Additional symptoms include weakness, trembling, and twitching of various muscles. The patient cannot drink even the smallest amount of wine.

Rhus toxicodendron (Poison ivy)

Rhus toxicodendron has proven successful in treating a constant

Although they may not know it, approximately 1 percent of the population suffers from the tormenting condition of restless legs.

urge to move around instead of lying still in bed. A feeling of stiffness or unease in the muscular system leads to an unconscious effort to find a comfortable position. In addition, the patient is often apprehensive at night.

Sciatica

Please also refer to "Lumbago."

Colocynthis (Bitter cucumber)

Treat shooting pains that follow insult, rage, or periodic spasmodic sciatic pain with *Colocynthis*. Typical symptoms include muscle cramps, numbness, and violent pains in the hip joint that feel as if it were being squeezed in a vise. The symptoms are worse with touch, with cold, with any arousal of emotion, and at night. They are relieved by hard pressure, drawing up the legs, lying on the painful side, rest, and warmth.

■ Dosage: 5 granules of *Colocynthis* twice a day

Gnaphalium (Cud weed)

You can treat shooting pains that stretch from the small of the back into the feet or the toes with *Gnaphalium*. The patient has a feeling of numbness in the affected areas. Both sides are involved, and they alternate. The symptoms are worse when lying down, at night, with exposure to damp cold, and with movement. You can relieve the pain by sitting up and by bending your knees.

■ Dosage: 5 granules of *Gnaphalium* 6C twice a day

Magnesium phosphoricum (Magnesium phosphate)

Use *Magnesium phosphoricum* to treat sciatic pains that come in spasms and shoot along the nerves. The symptoms are worse with light touch, with cold, and at night. They are relieved with pressure and warmth.

■ Dosage: 5 granules of *Magnesium phosphoricum* 12C twice a day

Physiotherapy can be very helpful in preventing recurring sciatic pain. These exercises stretch and relax the muscles of the back. In addition, you should train the abdominal muscles, too. Exercises using the Moshe Feldenkrais method are ideal because they are very gentle and very effective.

Valeriana (Valerian root)

Valeriana is effective in treating a sudden onset of shifting sciatic pain that feels like electric shocks and that alternates with nervousness and oversensitivity. The patient cannot sleep, and the insomnia often becomes worse when he takes medicines containing *Valeriana*. Resting, sitting, standing or stretching the affected leg aggravates the condition. Moving, walking, changing position, and relaxing the leg relieves the symptoms.

■ Dosage: 5 granules of *Valeriana* 6C twice a day

Shoulder Pain

Tearing pains in the shoulder caused by blows, falls, or rheumatic complaints can be relieved and cured with homeopathic remedies.

■ Dosage: 5 granules 6C (3 granules 12C of *Ferrum metallicum*) of the indicated remedy mornings and evenings; on improvement, 5 granules once a day

Arnica (Leopard's bane)

Use *Arnica* when the muscular system feels battered. The patient is afraid of being touched and wants to be left alone. The bed seems as hard as a rock. The symptoms are worse with touching, the slightest pressure, movement, or jarring. They improve when lying down, lowering the head, and resting.

Ferrum metallicum (Iron)

The pains in the left shoulder extend through the arm into the hand.

Ruta graveolens (Rue, Bitterwort)

Ruta can provide relief for bumps, blows, bruises, and for overexerted ligaments and tendons.

Important:
Do not use *Ruta* during pregnancy!

Bryonia (Wild hops, White bryony)

A treatment with *Bryonia* helps with shooting pains. It can ease the pain after overexertion, moving incorrectly, or getting chilled after physical exertion. The symptoms are worse with the slightest movement. They improve with rest, cool temperatures, lying on the painful area, or pressing hard on the painful spot.

Hypericum (St. John's wort)

Use *Hypericum* if *Arnica* does not produce the desired healing effect. The symptoms are worse with cold, dampness, fog, drafts, and touch. Bending the head backwards provides some relief.

Rhus toxicodendron (Poison ivy)

Rhus toxicodendron helps in cases of pulled ligaments and sprains. It works well when you have injured yourself lifting something heavy. It is known as the "moving man's remedy," and you can alternate using it and *Arnica*. The symptoms become worse at the beginning of any movement. Rest, wetness, and cold also aggravate the symptoms. Continued movement, warmth, and a hot-water bottle can provide relief.

Sprains, Strains

Strains and sprains occur suddenly. They can happen during sports, climbing the stairs, doing housework, or gardening. When you are in a hurry or are a little cold, your joints are susceptible to injuries such as painful strains and sprains.

Arnica (Leopard's bane)

In case of an accident in the house or garden, the first remedy to try is *Arnica*. It is the general remedy for trauma and overstraining. We also use it to treat problems that affect the whole body, such as hangover, weariness, and overexertion. Use *Arnica* specifically for exhaustion. The patient feels battered. He is afraid of being touched and behaves in a standoffish fashion. The bed seems rock hard. His head is hot, and his body is cold. The condition is worse with touch, even the slightest pressure. Movement

Rhus toxicodendron relieves pain in the shoulder that appears after exposure to a draft.

and jarring aggravate the symptoms. Improvement occurs when the patient is lying down, keeping his head low, and resting.

■ Dosage: 3 granules of *Arnica* 6C every half hour until the symptoms subside (for children give 2 granules 6C); it is also possible to take 2 or 3 granules 30C or 200C, but only once or twice a day

Bryonia (Wild hops, White bryony)

Shooting pains are a characteristic symptom indicating the use of *Bryonia*. It is useful if your back or other muscles ache after overexertion. The afflicted muscles are stiff and ache. The symptoms are worse with the slightest movement, warmth, or touch. They improve with resting, cool temperatures, lying on the painful area, or hard pressure on the affected spot.

■ Dosage: 3 granules of *Bryonia* 6C three times a day

Rhus toxicodendron (Poison ivy)

We call *Rhus toxicodendron* the "moving man's remedy." It relieves all symptoms of strains, sprains, overexertion, and injuries caused by heavy lifting. You can also alternate *Rhus toxicodendron* with *Arnica*. The condition is worse at night, when resting, or with wet and cold. Typically, the pain is worse at the beginning of every movement. It feels better with continued movement and with warmth.

■ Dosage: 5 granules of *Rhus toxicodendron* 6C two to three times a day for the first few days; then once a day; in combination with *Arnica*, alternate 3 granules 6C of each remedy every hour; after improvement, 5 granules of each once a day

Stomachache

If the stomachache persists over a period of time, your doctor or practitioner should rule out the possibility of an ulcer or tumor before you begin medicating yourself.

Strains and sprains almost always result in a swelling of the joint. This swelling persists for about three days, but it should ease off after about two weeks. You should see a specialist if you feel that the joint is dislocated, if putting weight on the joint is extremely painful, or if the pain is still increasing after the first few days.

Nux vomica (Poison nut)

Take *Nux vomica* to relieve a nervous or irritated stomach caused by excessive consumption of stimulants such as alcohol, coffee, nicotine, and drugs. The symptoms may also be the result of serious problems at work or of a chronic lack of exercise. Typical symptoms are a full and heavy feeling in the stomach after meals, a stomachache radiating in various directions, and painful burping with a sour or bitter taste. The symptoms are worse in the morning, one or two hours after eating, and after drinking alcohol or coffee. They improve in the evenings, with warmth, and with rest.

■ Dosage: 5 granules of *Nux vomica* 6C twice a day

Pulsatilla (Wind flower)

Severe emotional stress and bad eating habits, such as eating too quickly, eating foods that are too fatty, and eating meals that are too large often lead to stomach upsets and indigestion.

When the stomach upset begins after eating indiscriminately, after eating fatty or fried food, or after eating too much ice, you should use *Pulsatilla*. Typically, although the mouth is dry, the patient isn't thirsty. He has a nasty taste in his mouth after sour burps. Warm drinks seem to induce more vomiting than cold ones. The patient vomits food that was eaten a long time ago. The symptoms are worse in warm rooms. They improve with fresh air and with small amounts of ice.

■ Dosage: 5 granules of *Pulsatilla* 6C twice a day

Antimonium crudum (Crude antimony)

Typically, the patient has a strong desire for acids, sour wine, fruit, vinegar, and onions, but these make him vomit. *Antimonium* is also suitable for children who vomit after consuming milk and acids. Vomiting does not relieve the pain, and the tongue is coated white, as if painted. The patient is peevish. Hot water causes diarrhea. Burps taste of undigested food. The symptoms are worse after meals, with pastry, and with sour food. The symptoms improve with rest and with damp warmth.

■ Dosage: 3 granules of *Antimonium crudum* 12C twice a day

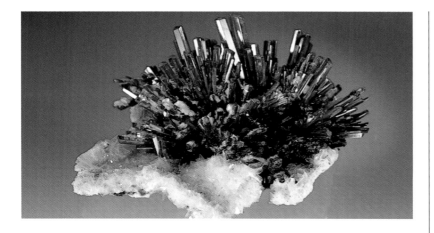

Antimony, a gray, brittle metal, is also called sulphide of antimony. It provides the source material for the homeopathic medicine, Antimonium crudum.

Sunburn

Roasting in the blazing sun for hours on end is no longer in fashion. Even a few minutes of exposure in southern areas can be dangerous for people with fair skin. Apart from the well-tried homeopathic medicines, you can find very effective creams, such as *Calendula* cream, Combudoron gel or liquid, and Dr. Bach's Rescue Cream.

Ferrum phosphoricum (Ferrum phosphate)

Ferrum phosphoricum is suitable in cases of light sunburn. In addition, cold compresses on the head can provide relief.

■ Dosage: 3 granules of *Ferrum phosphoricum* 12C every two hours

Belladonna (Deadly nightshade)

Use *Belladonna* if the skin is bright red. Other symptoms include dilated pupils, a reddened throat, and often a splitting headache.

■ Dosage: 5 granules of *Belladonna* 6C every two hours

Glonoinum (Nitroglycerin)

Glonoinum has proved successful in serious cases of sunburn with headache. The head feels too large. The patient can feel his heartbeat in his head or ears.

To relieve acute sunburn, first put on moist compresses using Combudoron (Weleda) or Rescue Lotion. A few hours later, apply a thin coating of *Combuduron* gel.

71

Do not underestimate the effects of the sun on a cloudy day. Even when the sky is overcast, your skin can burn in only a few minutes, especially in southern areas. In any area, if you stay unprotected in the sun for more than half an hour, you run the risk of sunburn.

■ Dosage: 5 granules of *Glonoinum* 6C every two hours

Cantharis (Spanish fly)

Cantharis works well when there are blisters, but it is also effective against any other type of burn in which the blisters have become inflamed.
■ Dosage: 5 granules of *Cantharis* 6C every two hours

Sunstroke

With sunstroke, your skin is hot and dry, you feel sick, drowsy, and sometimes feverish. Excessive thirst, vomiting, and diarrhea are also possible. Don't immediately retire to a cold room because your body must get used to the change in temperature gradually. Damp compresses on the forehead are helpful. Drink water slowly. If possible, add a little salt or sugar to the water. The following homeopathic remedies produce relief.
■ Dosage: 3 granules 6C of the indicated remedy every hour until improvement is noticed

Glonoinum (Nitroglycerin)

Use *Glonoinum* if you have a violent throbbing in the head, in the heart region, or in the chest (do not use *Belladonna* for these symptoms). The face is red or pale. The symptoms are worse with warmth and stooping. They improve with cold applications to the face.

Belladonna (Deadly nightshade)

Belladonna helps if the head is hot and the hands are cold. Typical symptoms are a bright red, hot face, dilated pupils, cold hands and feet, throbbing and visibly pulsating arteries at the temples and neck. The symptoms are worse with jarring, noise, light, and movement. They improve when the patient is covered up, leaning back, and resting.

First Aid for Sunstroke

- First, move the patient into the shade or into a cool room.
- Elevate the upper part of the body.
- Open tight clothing, belt, and tie.
- Cool the forehead and the back of the neck with damp compresses.
- Give small sips of cool drinks.
- If you don't notice improvement after five minutes or if the patient is unconscious, call an ambulance.

Aconite (Monk's hood)

Use *Aconite* if the patient feels ill, his face is deathly pale, and the blood in his head pulsates violently. Typically, the patient feels sick when he tries to get up. The headache feels better after he urinates.

Gelsemium (Yellow jasmine)

Gelsemium is the proper remedy if the patient is trembling and feels weak. The eyelids are so painful they can hardly be kept open. A numbing headache begins at the nape of the neck or at the back of the head and moves to the forehead and the eyes. The symptoms improve after urinating.

Apis (Honeybee)

Give *Apis* if the skin is taut and the neck is stiff. A bloated face and rosy skin are important indications for using *Apis*. You can also use *Apis* for children who have symptoms such as burrowing their heads into pillows or rocking their heads back and forth. Children may scream in their sleep. There is a great sensitivity to the slightest touch. The symptoms are worse with warmth and improve with cold.

Melilotus (Sweet clover)

Use *Melilotus* for an intolerable headache that pounds with every

Playing volleyball, tennis, golf, and other sports in the blazing sun without a hat is not only out of fashion but also extremely dangerous. The effects of the sun's rays combined with the increased brain circulation during exercise can lead to an irritation of the meninges (the membranes that surround the brain) and to sunstroke.

A stiff neck and the desire to keep the head bent back are indications that the meninges are involved. Bending the head forward leads to violent pain, which the patient will seek to avoid.

beat of the pulse. The patient has a bright red face and is often confused. The condition improves after he urinates.

Veratrum album (White hellebore)

Veratrum album helps in cases of sunstroke accompanied by vomiting and a feeling of extreme weakness. Additional indications are cold sweats and a strong desire for fresh air.

Tendinitis

Athletes aren't the only people who suffer from tendinitis. People who knit a lot, play the piano, or type also suffer from this ailment.

■ Dosage: 5 granules 6C of the indicated remedy twice a day (5 granules three times a day for *Symphytum* 4C) until improvement

Arnica (Leopard's bane)

Try this remedy as the first countermeasure. Usually, the symptoms are worse with touch, movement, jarring, damp, and cold. They improve with rest and with warmth.

Rhus toxicodendron (Poison ivy)

The best indication for using this remedy is that the symptoms seem to be better with continued movement, but the onset of each movement causes violent pain. The symptoms are worse in wet or cold weather. They improve with warmth and warm applications.

Tendinitis usually appears some time after a strain. If swelling or pain occurs while overstraining, you should consult an orthopedist or homeopath.

Bryonia (Wild hops, White bryony)

Bryonia is the remedy to use if the inflamed joint is hot and swollen. The slightest motion aggravates the symptoms. Exerting pressure on the painful area provides relief. Remaining still also helps.

Symphytum (Comphrey)

Symphytum aids the healing process when the symptoms include tingling, pricking pains. The symptoms are worse with pressure, touch, or motion. The patient feels better with warmth.

Nux vomica (Poison nut)

Use *Nux vomica* for inflammations in the left arm caused by a chill or draft. When the patient is stressed, the symptoms appear more frequently. The symptoms are worse with cold, in drafts, and with nervous tension. They improve when covered up, and with warmth, rest, and sleep.

Belladonna (Deadly nightshade)

Typically, the pain appears suddenly and vanishes just as suddenly. The swelling is red and hot, and the patient is indignant and angry.

Sore Throat

We recommend warm or cold throat compresses, depending on which temperature feels better on the throat.

Belladonna (Deadly nightshade)

Treat with *Belladonna* if the tonsils and throat are bright red and swollen. Often the right side feels worse than the left, and the sore throat starts suddenly, sometimes caused by cold air. The mouth is disagreeably dry. Despite the burning sensation in the throat, the patient feels a compulsion to swallow. He craves cold drinks, which only aggravate the complaints. The condition feels worse with cold compresses, swallowing, and speaking.

- Dosage: 3 granules of *Belladonna* 6C every hour; on improvement, increase the intervals

If you have a sore throat, decide whether cold or warm drinks relieve the symptoms. In addition, you can apply warm or cold compresses on your throat. Spread ricotta cheese or table salt on the compress.

Apis mellifica (Honeybee)

The tonsils, throat, and palate are glassy, swollen, and pale red. The patient feels a burning, stinging pain. The uvula is swollen like a bulging sack. Although the mouth is dry, the patient is not thirsty. The condition is worse with warmth, pressure, or touch. The patient feels better with cold or cold applications.

■ Dosage: 3 granules of *Apis* 6C every two hours

Hepar sulphuris (Calcium sulphide)

First, the throat becomes cold, and then it feels very sore. The tonsils are covered with pustules. The patient has the sensation that there is a splinter or fishbone stuck in his throat. The pain radiates into the ear when the patient yawns or turns his head. He is irritable and very sensitive to cold. The condition is aggravated by cold, cold drinks, and by uncovering the throat. The patient feels better with warmth, with warm applications, and in humid weather.

■ Dosage: 3 granules of *Hepar sulphuris* 12C every two to three hours

---

If the throat remains sore for several days with a high temperature and a coating of pus, you should consult your doctor or homeopath.

Phytolacca (Pokeweed)

Use *Phytolacca* when the tonsils and pharynx appear dark red and inflamed. The patient has shooting pains, usually on the right side, which radiate to his ears on swallowing. In addition, there are rheumatic pains and an exhausted, weak condition. The sore throat is usually caused by cold, damp weather. Warm drinks, pressure, or touch make the condition worse, and the symptoms are worse at night. Cold drinks relieve the pain.

■ Dosage: 3 granules of *Phytolacca* 6C every two to three hours

Travel Sickness

Be prepared for travel anxiety and motion sickness by putting together your own little homeopathic first-aid kit. See also "Diarrhea" and "Stomachache."

Aconite (Monk's hood)

Use *Aconite* when travel anxiety manifests itself with heart palpitations and a fear of flying. *Aconite* is also a reliable remedy for any shock or fear of traveling caused by an accident.

■ Dosage: 3 granules of *Aconite* 30C on the day before departure and half an hour before leaving

Coffea (Coffee)

In cases where nervous excitement, restlessness, or heart palpitations disturb the preparations for a journey, use *Coffea*. Do not drink coffee after taking *Coffea*.

■ Dosage: 3 granules of *Coffea* 30C on the day before departure and half an hour before leaving

Cocculus (Indian cockle)

Use *Cocculus* for problems with jet lag or nausea and vomiting along with giddiness and weakness. Typical symptoms suggesting the use of *Cocculus* are extreme sadness with the feeling that time is going by too quickly. The symptoms are worse with lack of sleep. They improve when lying down.

■ Dosage: before departure, take 3 granules of *Cocculus* 30C one to three times; on arrival, another 3 granules one to three times; in case of motion sickness, 3 granules of *Cocculus* 6C every half hour

Petroleum (Crude rock oil)

If you have a constant feeling of sickness as long as the vehicle is

Tabacum (Tobacco) relieves motion sickness when the symptoms are pale or yellow-green skin, cold sweat, and a profuse flow of saliva. The patient feels awful and has to close his eyes while the vehicle is in motion. The symptoms are worse with warmth, with the eyes open, and with tobacco smoke. Fresh air and loosening the clothes provide relief. Dosage: 3 granules of *Tabacum* 6C every half hour.

What Is Travel Sickness?

Travel Anxiety

Even before beginning the journey, fear and excitement are stressful, affecting sleep, the general well-being, and the entire nervous system.

Motion Sickness

Motion sickeness develops because the organ in the inner ear that regulates balance cannot adapt to the motion of the car, bus, ship, or plane.

in motion, the correct remedy is *Petroleum*. In spite of the sickness, the patient is hungry. A feeling of dizziness occurs.

■ Dosage: 3 granules of *Petroleum* 6C every half hour

Voice Loss

Sometimes with a cough or hoarseness, the patient can only croak or whisper. In extreme cases, the patient may even lose his voice completely. The following remedies can relieve or even cure the symptoms.

■ Dosage: 3 granules 6C (12C for *Ferrum phosphoricum*) of the indicated remedy two to three times a day

Bromium (Bromium)

Treat with *Bromium* when the loss of voice is preceded by a cough, diarrhea, or asthma after warm days with cool evenings. A person who needs *Bromium* sweats easily with exertion and is then very sensitive to cooling down or to drafts. When he breathes, he makes a rattling noise, and he has a dry, spasmodic, wheezing cough. The patient feels that the air he is inhaling is cold. The condition becomes worse when inhaling cold air and in warm rooms. Cold drinks provide some relief. The patient does well at the seashore.

Arum maculatum (Cuckoo-pint)

After exposure to dry cold, *Arum* relieves the tickling and itching that occur in the nose, the larynx, and on the lips.

Phosphorus (Phosphorus)

Use *Phosphorus* in cases of a hard, dry cough.

Arum triphyllum (Jack-in-the-pulpit)

When a great amount of mucus is discharged and spat out, use *Arum triphyllum*.

■ *Aconite* helps if the voice is about to fail after exposure to dry cold.
■ *Ferrum phosphoricum* is the remedy for speakers, singers, and anyone who tends to overexert his voice.
■ *Ignatia* helps patients with overstrained voices who often sigh and wail.
■ *Gelsemium* is helpful if the loss of voice sets in after menstruation.

Vomiting

In cases of vomiting, we recommend sipping water or tepid herbal tea so that the body does not become dehydrated. If vomiting continues for longer than a day, you should consult your doctor or practitioner.

Nux vomica (Poison nut)

Use *Nux vomica* for complaints that occur after anger, overeating, too much alcohol, late-night meals, and light poisoning with chemicals. The symptoms include retching with an ineffectual urge to vomit. Also use *Nux vomica* for vomiting when hawking up mucus. The patient is irritable and finds fault with everything. The symptoms are worse after eating, drinking, and moving.

■ Dosage: 5 granules of *Nux vomica* 6C every two hours

Arsenicum album (Arsenic trioxide, White arsenic)

Use *Arsenicum album* in cases of diarrhea and sickness that occur after eating food that has gone bad or that is infected with salmonellae or after eating ice cream. The sickness can occur in spasms or after eating and drinking. The smell of food alone causes nausea. The patient is very thirsty but only drinks in small sips. A feeling of weakness and cold sweats makes him want to lie down, but anxiety and restlessness prevent him from relaxing or sleeping. The condition is worse after midnight, when moving, eating, or drinking even small amounts of water.

■ Dosage: 3 granules of *Arsenicum album* 12C every hour

Ipecacuanha (Root of ipecac)

Use *Ipecacuanha* in cases of continued sickness after anger, after eating ice cream, and with headache and persistent nausea. Additional symptoms include a profuse flow of saliva and a moist tongue with no coating. The condition is worse when the patient bends down.

■ Dosage: 5 granules of *Ipecacuanha* 6C every two hours

Use *Aethusa* (Fool's parsley) to help babies or infants who vomit violently after drinking their mother's milk and then go on drinking. It is also effective in sudden onsets of violent sickness in the heat of summer. The patient is very weak, has a gaunt face, and suffers from cold sweats. Dosage: 5 granules of *Aethusa* 6C three times a day.

Weather Sensitivity

Old people are not the only ones who suffer from weather-related complaints. School children also have difficulties concentrating when the weather changes or when it is very hot. Complaints related to the weather frequently disturb the general well-being and produce headaches or circulatory problems.

■ Dosage: 5 granules 6C of the indicated remedy twice a day

Rhododendron (Siberian rhododendron)

Rhododendron is the best remedy for headache and rheumatic pain caused by a change in the weather. The symptoms are especially severe before or during a period of stormy weather. The patient experiences relief when the storm has died down, or with warmth.

Natrium muriaticum (Sodium chloride, Table salt)

When the weather turns hot, use *Natrium muriaticum* to cure your weather-related symptoms. This remedy is also good for cold sores caused by sunbathing in mountainous areas and by allergies to the sun. *Natrium muriaticum* is the appropriate remedy for rashes that occur while you are vacationing at the seaside.

Natrium sulphuricum (Sodium sulphate)

This remedy is especially effective if you are easily exhausted in hot, humid weather. Rheumatic pain often occurs when the weather is cold and wet. *Natrium sulphuricum* is the appropriate remedy for this, too.

Natrium carbonicum (Sodium carbonate)

Treat headache and giddiness that arise after extreme exertion in the midday heat with *Natrium carbonicum*. The patient has a tendency to dislocate or sprain his ankles easily.

Even if weather sensitivity is a disagreeable complaint, look on the positive side: Your body is responding to its environment and to nature. Being a "weatherman" often produces a feeling of enthusiasm once the symptoms have eased off.

The 31 Most Important Remedies

What follows is an alphabetical list with short explanations of the most important homeopathic remedies. The descriptions list the symptoms that indicate the use of the remedy and describe the patient's appearance and physical and mental condition. For the dosages for each ailment and for further homeopathic remedies, you should look up the appropriate ailment in the section on "Ailments from A to Z."

Aconitum napellus, Aconite (Monk's hood)

Violent, severe complaints appear suddenly, accompanied by a high temperature. The symptoms are caused by an emotional shock or by a shock resulting from a sudden drop in temperature with cold, dry air. Characteristic symptoms include a loss of strength, excessive restlessness, fearfulness, and a fear of dying. A fever that responds to *Aconite* usually begins at night, shortly after the patient goes sleep. The fever is accompanied by severe chills. The temperature rises to over 104° F (40° C). The skin and mucous membranes are hot and dry. The patient exhibits restlessness and fearfulness and has heart palpitations with a strong, rapid pulse. His face is red, but it becomes pale when he sits up. The patient wants cold drinks.

Allium cepa (Red onion)

Allium cepa is used to treat a constant dripping nose, an acrid secretion of the nose which makes the nostrils and upper lip sore, and a mild flow of tears that burns the eyes.

 In cold, damp weather, *Allium cepa* cures a cold with hoarseness, a dry cough that causes a tickling irritation in the larynx, dif-

Modalities
The symptoms are worse at night and in the evening, in warm rooms, when lying on the affected side, and in cold winds. They improve outdoors and when sweating.

The common onion, Allium cepa, *has a beautiful spherical flower.*

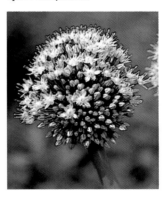

ficulties in breathing due to a feeling of pressure in the middle of the chest, headache, and a feeling of heat accompanied by thirst.

Apis mellifica (Honeybee)

Characteristic symptoms for using *Apis mellifica* are a swelling and inflammation with sticking pains and extreme sensitivity to heat, touch, and pressure from clothing. Additional symptoms include a fiery red, swollen, painful tongue that often occurs in combination with a cold spot on the tip of the nose. The patient is listless, drowsy, jealous, nervous, and cries out in his sleep.

■ You can use *Apis mellifica* for a sore throat with extremely swollen and pink tonsils and pharynx. The uvula is puffed up and elongated and has a baglike appearance. It is also helpful for inflammation of the middle ear that gets worse with the application of warmth, for insect bites and bee stings, for fever that is not accompanied by thirst and a desire to uncover oneself, and for severe swelling of the upper eyelids and lachrymal sacs.

Arnica montana (Leopard's bane)

Arnica is the first remedy to use with all blunt injuries such as bruises, strains, crushing injuries, hematomas, and aching muscles.

■ Typical symptoms are a weariness of the body and limbs, especially when lying down, aches throughout the whole body, and a sensation that the bed is unbearably hard. Although the patient is overly tired, he has trouble falling asleep. He wants to be left alone, rejects the people who are treating him, behaves in a standoffish manner, and is afraid of being touched.

■ *Arnica* is useful after falls or dog bites, before giving birth, before operations, before a visit to the dentist, and with giddiness and high blood pressure. It is also useful for older people after a heart attack or a stroke and to prevent hemorrhages and embolisms.

Arsenicum album (Arsenic trioxide, White arsenic)

The patient is restless. Although he is thirsty, he only wants small sips of water. He suffers from burning pain and anxiety and a fear of death, especially after midnight and after extreme exhaustion.

■ *Arsenic* has proved effective in cases of severe sickness with diarrhea, food poisoning combined with feebleness, sickness after ice cream or milk (especially during pregnancy), and many skin diseases, including neurodermatitis.

Belladonna (Deadly nightshade)

Belladonna is used for diseases that appear suddenly. Usually these are accompanied by a high fever and a red face. The patient

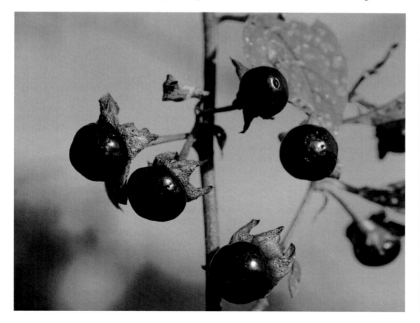

Modalities

The symptoms are worse after midnight, with cold, with the slightest exertion, after cold food and drink, and after milk. They improve after warm applications, with warm drinks, and in the fresh air.

Modalities

The symptoms are worse with touch, with summer sun, with noise, after midnight, and while drinking. They improve when resting, standing, or sitting.

The active substance of Atropa belladonna *is highly poisonous. You must never eat the berries or any other part of this plant. The active substance is only used in medicine and natural healing in a controlled, extreme dilution.*

steams under the bedclothes but does not want to be uncovered. With fever, there is no thirst, but otherwise the patient is very thirsty for cold water, has a dry mouth, and has no anxiety (unlike the symptoms indicating *Aconite*).

- *Belladonna* is the main remedy for scarlet fever. It is effective in cases of heatstroke, sunburn, and sciatic pains. You can use it to stimulate labor pains and to cure diseases caused by cold, damp weather and wet hair.

Bryonia alba (Wild hops, White bryony)

Bryonia is used when the mucous membranes (especially those in the nose and intestines) and the lips are extremely dry and there is a constant thirst for cold drinks. Severe constipation with dry, hard stools occurs. The patient is irritable, easily flies into a temper, wants to be left alone, and feels best at home.

- *Bryonia* is successful in curing headaches, complaints of the joints, and problems with digestion accompanied by coughing (if the other indicated symptoms are present).

Carbo vegetabilis (Vegetable charcoal)

Carbo vegetabilis is a good remedy for very low vitality. Typical symptoms are a tendency to faint, constant exhaustion, and an urge for fresh air.

- *Carbo vegetabilis* is good for collapse, weakness, and cold sweats. You can use it for food poisoning, flatulence, and with Roemheld Syndrome (the bloated intestines press against the diaphragm and thus cause heart complaints). It is also used successfully to cure varicose veins, especially during pregnancy.

Chamomilla (German chamomile)

This is the best remedy for restless, bad-tempered people and for children who always want to be carried around or keep

---

Modalities

The symptoms are worse with warmth and the smallest movement. They improve with damp weather, pressure on the painful spot, and rest.

Modalities

The symptoms are worse in the evening, at night, outdoors, and in the cold. Greasy food, butter, milk, and coffee aggravate the condition. The symptoms improve after burping.

Modalities

The symptoms are worse with heat, stress, and wind, and at night. They improve in warm, damp weather.

demanding toys and then throw them away.

■ *Chamomilla* is very suitable for teething babies and for intense, hot earaches that torture the patient. A typical symptom indicating the use of *Chamomilla* is one red cheek and one pale cheek.

China (Peruvian bark)

This remedy is successfully employed in convalescence after a large blood loss or after a lengthy bout of diarrhea with vomiting.

■ *China* is very useful for headaches in the face and for giddiness. It is also very suitable for treating diarrhea that appears after every meal, especially after eating fruit. *China* provides relief when foul-smelling flatulence fills the whole abdomen.

Modalities
The symptoms are worse with the slightest touch and after meals. They improve with doubling up, being outdoors, and being warm.

Ferrum phosphoricum (Ferrum phosphate)

■ *Ferrum phosphoricum* is a good remedy for use at the onset of a fever that comes on gradually. It has also proved successful at the onset of any inflammatory disease and for the early stage of earache. *Ferrum phosphoricum* is well suited for nervous, sensitive people who are easily exhausted.

Modalities
The symptoms are worse at night from 4 to 6 A.M. and when bumped or touched on the right side. They improve with applications of cold.

Gelsemium (Yellow jasmine)

■ *Gelsemium* is effective in relieving the results of fright, fear, excitement, and emotional agitation. It is a good remedy to take before an exam that you are afraid of or that is making you nervous.

■ *Gelsemium* works well against flu-like symptoms that begin slowly and are accompanied by a headache rising up from the back of the neck, by chattering teeth, and by a lack of thirst.

■ *Gelsemium* is also a good remedy for diarrhea that appears primarily after meals, for trembling weakness, exhaustion, chilliness, and the feeling that you have a band around your head.

Modalities
The symptoms are worse in the sun, with jarring, overheating, shaking, and with pressure from a headband. They improve with cold wrappings, cold air, and pressure.

Ignatia amara (St. Ignatius bean)

If you are suffering from homesickness, love sickness, or the loss of a loved one and your emotional balance is off, *Ignatia* is the correct remedy. It is often described as a women's remedy.

- Changeable moods, a tendency to paroxysms of laughter and crying, and frequent sighing and moaning are signs pointing to the use of *Ignatia*. In addition, *Ignatia* patients feel as if they have a lump in their throat, and they suffer from sleeplessness with a great deal of yawning.

Modalities

The symptoms are worse with tobacco, in smoky rooms, with a light touch, strong smells, and grief. They improve with a change of position, firm pressure, and warmth.

Kali bichromicum (Potassium bichromate)

- Typically, we use *Kali bichromicum* for diseases of the nose and mouth that are accompanied by a tough, sticky, yellow green discharge. Round, dot-shaped crusts in the nose are also typical. The tongue usually has a thick yellow coating. The patient's sense of smell is impaired.
- *Kali bichromicum* relieves the sudden onset of pain and sciatic complaints.

Modalities

The symptoms are worse after beer, in the mornings, and on days with warm, humid weather. They improve with heat.

Kali carbonicum (Potash, Potassium carbonate)

Kali carbonicum is a very effective remedy for stabbing pains that often appear in the lower right part of the chest.

- *Kali carbonicum* works well for dry, spasmodic coughs with retching and vomiting and for severe flatulence that plagues the patient after eating even a little food. It is also a remedy to stimulate labor.

Modalities

The symptoms are worse in the fresh air, in the early morning (especially from 2–5 A.M.), after exertion, and when lying on the left side. They improve in warm weather and with burping.

Lachesis (Bushmaster snake)

Lachesis is frequently used as a remedy for women during menopause. Primarily, it is employed in septic diseases caused by infections.

■ *Lachesis* is used for severe inflammations of the tonsils or the salivary glands when the symptoms begin on the left side and extend to the right. The feeling of having a lump in the throat also points to the use of *Lachesis*. The patient is overly sensitive to tight clothing. Wounds bleed profusely, and the blood is dark.

■ *Lachesis* helps patients who talk a lot and who are often too tired in the daytime to work. These people are usually suspicious and jealous.

Modalities
The symptoms are worse after sleeping, with tight clothing, and in humid warmth. They improve with the free discharge of secretions such as catarrh, sweat, or menstruation.

Ledum (Marsh tea)

Ledum is a good remedy for all bites and insect stings, especially bees. It is also used for puncture wounds caused by nails.

■ This is the remedy for rheumatic diseases without fever, such as arthritis and gout.

■ It helps in cases of animal bites, spiders' poison, and allergic reactions.

■ Coldness in the affected parts is a characteristic symptom indicating the use of *Ledum*.

Modalities
The symptoms are worse with warmth. They improve with cold.

Lycopodium (Club moss)

■ *Lycopodium* is regarded as a male remedy. The patient who suffers from intense flatulence in the lower bowels needs *Lycopodium* for relief. He is always ravenously hungry but is satisfied after a few mouthfuls.

■ The patient has an excessive desire for sweets. The symptoms usually begin on the right side and then move to the left.

■ *Lycopodium* is an important remedy for the liver because it is effective against all symptoms caused by a weak liver metabolism, such as flatulence and diarrhea, but also constipation, gout, rheumatic diseases, and even varicose veins.

Modalities
The symptoms are worse from 4–8 P.M. and in the morning. One foot or hand may be cold and the other warm. The symptoms improve outdoors and with warmth.

Magnesium phosphoricum (Magnesium phosphate)

Magnesium phosphoricum has an antispasmodic and pain-relieving effect in cases of abdominal spasms and intense flatulence. It relieves sudden violent paroxysms of shooting and sharp neuralgic pains, as well as menstrual cramps.

Mercurius solubilis (Mercury)

Mercurius relieves complaints in various parts of the body.
- Intestines: It is an important remedy for severe diarrhea and dysentery.
- Stomach: You may treat heartburn, foul burps, and chronic indigestion with *Mercurius*.
- Respiratory tract: Use when the cough is rough and dry, when the patient usually coughs twice at a time, and when he cannot lie on his right side.
- Mucous membranes of the mouth: Treat with *Mercurius* when the production of saliva increases primarily at night. The patient suffers from an offensive odor in the mouth and has a metallic taste in his mouth. This remedy produces good results in cases of spongy, receding gums and of canker sores on the tongue. There is an excessive thirst, although the mouth is moist.
- Teeth: Use this primarily for aches in the root of the tooth at night.
- Sinus: The nostrils are raw; sunshine causes sneezing. A middle ear infection often occurs on the right side.
- Head: The patient is sensitive to the weather or has a feeling of tension in the head.
- General: There is a tendency to slow healing, to septic and foul-smelling ulcers, to trembling hands, and to oily skin.

Natrium muriaticum
(Sodium chloride, table salt)

Natrium muriaticum works well in cases where prolonged problems, grief, and disappointment cause a disease.

■ People who need *Natrium muriaticum* want to be left alone to weep, but they can become very irritable if ignored. They do a lot for their community.

■ A *Natrium muriaticum* patient is drowsy in the daytime, especially after meals. In spite of a large appetite for food and drink, the patient is very thin, especially in the neck. He loves salty pretzels, salty meat, and spicy food. If he is constipated, his stool is dry. A typical symptom is that the patient cannot urinate in the presence of others.

■ This remedy is also very effective with headaches, migraines, bronchitis, colds, complaints of the digestive organs, and skin diseases.

Modalities

The symptoms are worse with anger, trouble, direct sunlight, noises, and sexual intercourse. They improve with fasting, tight clothing, and lying down. They also improve in the afternoon and at night.

Nux vomica (Poison nut)

Usually a male remedy, *Nux vomica* is especially suited for thin, active, nervous, stressed manager types who like to eat heavy meals which do not agree with them. They are often heavy smokers and coffee drinkers, and they suffer from a chronically dry mouth.

■ Use *Nux vomica* for cramps that appear with migraines, gastritis, duodenal ulcers, or spasmodic constipation. It relieves stomach disorders with heartburn and burping, a full feeling (one to three hours after meals), indigestion after meals that are too large and too greasy, and after an excess of alcohol, coffee, and nicotine. The patient often feels cold and catches a cold easily from cold and draft.

■ It also helps the menstrual complaints of women who hate their period because they "don't function" well at this time of the month.

Modalities

The symptoms are worse in the morning, with mental strain, after meals, and with drugs and stimulants. They improve at night, with rest, and after a nap.

Phosphorus (**Phosphorus**)

Phosphorus is suitable for sociable, warmhearted, and helpful people. These people are slender or even emaciated, and they are easily exhausted. Fair or reddish hair is characteristic, as is rapid growth in children and juveniles.

■ The *Phosphorus* type is afraid of the dark, of being alone, and of thunderstorms. He is easily exhausted but recovers his strength very quickly. He is especially sensitive to noises and to smells. He has a glowing, impressive charisma.

■ Use *Phosphorus* if the hands and feet burn or if the back burns from top to bottom. The pain can also appear between the shoulder blades. The patient cannot lie on the left side.

■ *Phosphorus* types often vomit food and drink as soon as it has reached the stomach. They are revolted by boiled milk and are very thirsty for cold drinks. Palpitation, heartburn, breathing difficulties, and hemorrhages from all organs are also possible. These people bruise easily.

Pulsatilla (**Wind flower**)

Pulsatilla is a typical remedy for women and children. It is effective for gentle, weepy, ginger-haired, girl-like women. These are mild and good-natured, but they can also be silly and mischievous. They are inconsistent and moody, especially when they are ill. Pulsatilla people can't bear to be alone; they love company and are very motherly.

■ Characteristic symptoms indicating the use of *Pulsatilla* are shifting and changeable complaints or a noticeable frequency of eye and ear diseases.

■ Mucous discharges are usually thick, mild, and creamy. *Pulsatilla* people have a desire for fresh air, but they feel chilly and have cold feet. Hot flushes, rapid changes of mood, and a strong tendency to varicose veins are also typical symptoms.

■ Indigestion occurs after greasy, heavy meals. The patient isn't very thirsty. *Pulsatilla* is an excellent remedy for stimulating labor. It has also proved effective in diseases that appear after getting wet, such as bladder problems.

Rhus toxicodendron (Poison ivy)

Rhus toxicodendron relieves all ailments caused by wet and cold.

■ It is useful for strains, sprains, and injuries which result from lifting. You can also use it after overexertion, for aching and stiff joints, for shoulder and arm problems, and for rheumatic pain due to cold and damp weather.

■ Characteristically, the pain increases at the beginning of movement and improves with continued movement. We also use *Rhus toxicodendron* as a remedy for neuralgia, sciatic and face pains, for burning, itching rashes with blisters, for influenza with aching limbs, and for a dry, tickling cough.

Modalities
The symptoms are worse during sleep, at night, at rest, with cold, and with wetness. They are better with continued movement (although they feel worse at the onset of movement), with warm applications, in warm weather, and when sweating.

Sepia (Cuttlefish ink)

Sepia is an important female remedy. The classic *Sepia* woman is slender with dark hair. She appears worn-out and has poor posture. She often has cold hands and feet and is easily cold. She is critical and distrustful and wants to be left on her own. The *Sepia* has no great desire for family and sex. Independence is very important to her. She has a tendency to depression.

Ruta graveolens (Rue, Bitterwort)

■ *Ruta graveolens* is useful for all crushings, strains, bruises, injuries of the periosteum, and pain in the tendons.

■ Use it also for tendinitis, tennis elbow, and muscle rheumatism.

■ If your eyes are overstrained from watching too much TV or working at the computer, *Ruta* relieves the ensuing headache, the burning, and the feeling of heat.

Modalities
The symptoms are worse in the evening, in cold and damp weather, after stooping, and lifting. They are better when moving, with warmth, and when lying on the back.

■ The *Sepia* woman hates housekeeping but is always worrying about it. If she makes a timid endeavor to break out of her rut, she runs off on a long walk all alone.

■ *Sepia* cures nervous disorders, menstrual complaints, and pains during menopause with hot flushes and sweating.

■ *Sepia* is also successful in dealing with sickness and vomiting that appear at the sight of certain foods, for instance during pregnancy. Take it if you have an empty feeling in the stomach, even right after meals.

■ Use *Sepia* in cases of chronic gastroenteritis, varicose veins, and hemorrhoids combined with hormonal disorders.

■ Additionally, you can use *Sepia* if you are experiencing a sensation of bearing down in the bladder, difficulties in retaining urine, or a feeling that the uterus is being dragged down. *Sepia* is a good remedy for constipation when you feel a ball in the rectum. It is also useful for itching, dry, or blistering rashes. In men, it relieves prostatitis.

Modalities

The symptoms are worse during rest, before and during menstruation, in crowded or stuffy rooms, with dampness, and after sweating. They are better with intense exercise and after hot applications.

Silicea (Silica, Pure flint, Rock crystal, Quartz)

Silicea is for timid and cautious people. These people have a chronic chilliness with cold hands and cold feet. *Silicea* types have extraordinarily good memories, but they often take a long time to finish a piece of work because they always see something they want to improve. They are soft, indecisive, and often very jumpy.

■ A typical symptom is cold sweat on the head and feet. This makes the skin on the soles and between the toes feel sore and smell bad. *Silicea* people fear pointed objects. They are oversensitive to noises. *Silicea* children are shy and fearful; they need their mother's encouragement. Often they don't thrive properly.

■ This remedy is also useful for all suppurations of the skin, nails, and hair, for a stuffy nose with loss of smell, and for dry crusts in the nose.

■ *Silicea* is also a remedy for constipation with the feeling that

Modalities

The symptoms are worse with drafts and cold, when bareheaded, with fresh air and exercise, at night, and on lying down. They are better when wrapped up warm and with warmth in general. Stomach upsets improve with cold food.

the stool is receding. It helps relieve headaches that begin at the back of the neck and extend to the eyes.

Sulphur **(Sublimated sulphur)**

Outwardly, the *Sulphur* type appears unkempt. He loves old clothes that he wears again and again. His hair is dull and tousled. The *Sulphur* person is stubborn and selfish but quite sociable. He can walk for hours, but he can't bear standing for a long time. He sticks his hot feet out of bed at night or uncovers himself completely.

■ A great feeling of weakness occurs at about 11 A.M., and he has to have something to eat. He is ravenous. If a *Sulphur* person has to go on a diet, he suffers from headaches. He craves sweets. The person is energetic and industrious, but then he suddenly develops an aversion to his job. He wakes up often during the night, and the slightest noise disturbs him. Typical

Modalities
The symptoms are worse at 11 A.M., when standing, in the warmth of bed, from water, and in warm rooms. They are better with movement, dry weather, and when lying on the right side.

The chemical element Sulphur *is not a metal. It crystalizes to a yellow, brittle formation. This is a* Sulphur *crystal on calcite.*

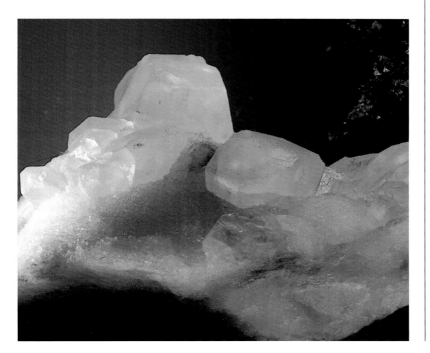

symptoms are dry skin and brittle hair. There is a tendency to skin diseases that itch.

■ *Sulphur* is the medicine that often helps if the patient doesn't respond to other homeopathic remedies. It has a very wide range and is important for old people. *Sulphur* is a remedy for acute and chronic enteritis, constipation, and hemorrhoids, if the modalities are right. It is also used for burning pains, acne, eczema, boils, varicose veins, and asthma.

Thuja occidentalis (Arbor vitae, Tree of life)

In Hahnemann's time, *Thuja* was the main remedy for gonorrhea. Today, it relieves many symptoms derived from this disease.

■ We use *Thuja* for skin rashes if they appear on parts covered with clothing. It is also helpful in dealing with various forms of warts and with cracked and brittle nails and with soft and peeling nails. *Thuja* helps with all the reactions to vaccination.

■ You can combat chronic cystitis and a burning sensation during urination with *Thuja* if there is the characteristic feeling that some urine was left in the urethra after urinating. For men, this is a remedy for inflammation and enlargement of the prostate gland.

Veratrum album (White hellebore)

Veratrum album is an excellent remedy for sudden circulatory collapse with cold sweat.

■ It is used for sickness with vomiting and diarrhea, acute food poisoning, summer diarrhea, or extreme weakness after every bowel movement. The patient is totally feeble, and the tip of his nose is ice cold.

Modalities
The symptoms are worse with dampness and cold, while stretching, after vaccination, and with constant tea drinking. They are better when resting, in warmth, in fresh air, and by bending the limbs.

Modalities
The symptoms are worse with movement, after drinking, and during or after bowel movement. They are better with pressure on the crown of the head.

Index of Remedies

acidum carbolicum, 54
acidum nitricum, 25 – 26
acidum phosphoricum, 62
acidum sulphuricum, 26
aconite, 3, 30, 34, 41, 45, 46, 62, 65, 73,
  76 – 77, 78, 81
aesculus, 54
aethusa, 79
allium cepa, 3, 26, 81 – 82
alumen, 31
ammonium carbonicum, 64
antimonium crudum, 70, 71
apis mellifica, 3, 19, 20, 30, 42, 56, 58, 73,
  75 – 76, 82
arnica montana, 3, 19, 23, 51, 58, 60, 63,
67, 68 – 69, 74, 82
arsenicum album, 3, 10, 11, 24, 28, 38,
  39, 65, 79, 83
arum maculatum, 78
arum triphyllum, 78
atropa belladonna, 4, 83
atropinum sulphuricum, 50
belladonna, 3, 14, 23, 28, 33, 42, 45 – 46,
  71, 72, 75, 83 – 84
bellis perennis, 19
berberis, 21
borax, 25
bromium, 36, 78
bryonia alba, 3, 31, 33, 34, 61, 67 – 68,
  69, 74, 84
cocculus, 77
caladium, 58
calcium carbonicum, 18, 64
calendula, 22 – 23, 25, 58, 71
cantharis, 20 – 21, 24, 72
capsicum, 56, 64
carbo vegetabilis, 3, 47, 52, 54, 56, 84
causticum, 24, 56
cedron, 22
chamomilla, 3, 38, 42 – 43, 45, 56, 59,
  84 - 85
chelidonium, 22, 51
china, 3, 17, 32, 40, 41, 47 – 48, 85
cinchona pubescens, 41
cinchona succirubra, 41

citrullus colocynthis, 13
clay, healing, 14, 53
coffea, 45, 59, 77
colocynthis, 12 – 13, 50, 66
Combudoron, 23, 71
conium, 20, 36 – 37
drosera, 35
dulcamara, 21
echinacea angustifolia, 26, 28, 29
eupatorium perfoliatum, 49
euphrasia, 26 – 27, 29
ferrum metallicum, 67
ferrum phosphoricum, 3, 23, 30, 43, 46,
  71, 78, 85
fever, 45 – 46
gelsemium, 3, 43, 49, 73, 78, 85
glonoinum, 71, 72
gnaphalium, 66
graphites, 44, 64
hamamelis, 23 – 24, 25, 55
hepar sulphuris, 14, 16 – 17, 33, 44, 76
hyoscyamus niger, 3, 37 – 38
hypericum, 58, 63, 68
ignatia amara, 3, 17, 59, 78, 86
ipecacuanha, 34, 40, 79
iris versicolor, 53
juglans regia, 16
kali bichromicum, 3
kali bromatum, 16, 62, 65
kali carbonicum, 3, 86
lachesis, 3, 86 – 87
ledum, 3, 58, 87
luffa, 27
lycopodium, 3, 18, 21, 32, 47, 53 – 54, 87
magnesium phosphoricum, 3, 12, 13, 50,
  52, 54, 62 – 63, 66, 88
melilotus, 73 – 74
mercurius solubilis, 3, 25, 57, 88
mezereum, 63
myristica sebifera, 14
natrium carbonicum, 80
natrium muriaticum, 3, 30 – 31, 80, 89
natrium sulphuricum, 80
nux moschata, 45, 52
nux vomica, 3, 12, 22, 32, 39, 45, 48, 51,

  52, 53, 54 – 55, 56, 60, 60 – 61, 70,
  75, 79, 89
paeonia, 55
petroleum, 77 – 78
phosphorus, 3, 35, 78, 90
phytolacca americana, 56, 76
plumbum metallicum, 32
podophyllum, 39 – 40
propolis, 25
pulsatilla, 3, 11, 21, 22, 27, 29, 38,
  39, 42, 45, 50 – 51, 52, 56 – 57,
  70, 90 – 91
Rescue Remedy, Bach's, 58, 71
rhododendron, 80
rhus toxicodendron, 3, 19, 30, 44,
  48, 49, 57, 60, 65 – 66, 68, 69,
  74, 91
robinia pseudoacacia, 52, 53
ruta graveolens, 3, 29, 67, 91
St. John's - wort oil, 19
sambucus, 27, 56
selenium, 15
sempervivum, 25
sepia, 3, 11, 29 – 30, 91 – 92
silicea, 3, 14, 15 – 16, 16 – 17, 56,
  92 – 93
sinapis nigra, 22
solanum tuberosum, 18
spongia, 35 – 36
staphisagria, 58
sticta pulmonaria, 37
sulphur, 3, 16, 17, 43, 93 – 94
symphytum, 74, 74 – 75
tabacum, 77
taraxacum, 22
tea trea oil, 58
teucrium, 22
thuja occidentalis, 3, 31
tormentilla, 25
urtica urens, 24
valeriana, 62, 67
veratrum album, 3, 39, 74, 94
vincetoxicum, 28
zincum metallicum, 65
zincum valerianium, 61

Subject Index

abdominal pains, 12 – 13
abscess, 13 – 15
acne, 15 – 16, 94
appetite disorders, 17, 18
backache, 18 – 20
bad breath, 22
bladder inflammation, 20 – 21
bleeding gums, 51
bronchitis cough, 32 – 36
burns, 22 – 24
canker sores, 25 – 26
catarrh, 26 – 28
centesimal potencies, 8, 9, 10
clay, healing, 14, 53
colds, 28
compresses, 27, 34, 40, 46, 63, 71, 72, 75, 82
conjunctivitis, 28 – 31
constipation, 12, 31 – 32, 32, 89, 92 – 93, 94
constitutional medicine, 11
coughs, 36, 78, 84
cravings during pregnancy, 18
cystitis, 20, 21, 94
decimal potencies (X or D), 8, 9, 10
depression, 59, 91
diarrhea, 32, 38 – 40, 41, 72, 78, 94
dosage, 9
earache, 41 – 43
eczema, 43 – 44, 94
examination, homeopathic, 6
fainting, 44 – 45, 84
fever, 45 – 46
flatulence, 12, 47 – 48, 48, 50, 54
flu-like symptoms, 48 – 49
gallbladder problems, 50 – 51
Hahnemann, Samuel, 6, 7, 8, 51, 94
hay fever, 27
heartburn, 12, 52 – 54
hemorrhoids, 39, 54 – 55, 92, 94
hoarseness, 55 – 57
insect bites and stings, 58

kidney inflammation, 12, 20 – 21
law of similars, 4, 7
LM potencies, 8, 9, 10
lumbago, 60
meningitis, 41, 73, 74
menstruation, 12, 13, 22, 54, 78, 86, 89, 92
modalities, 10, 81 – 95
mother tincture, 7, 8, 22 – 23, 58
mucous membranes, mouth, 25, 88
nervous disorders, 61 – 62
nervousness, 65 – 66
neuralgia, 62 – 63
onion bag, 42
overweight, 63 – 64
potentization, 7, 9 – 10
poultice, 14
pregnancy, 54, 67, 84, 92
principle of similarity, 6, 7
principles of homeopathy, 7
prostate, 94
Q potencies, 8
quantum theory, 9
restless legs, 65, 66
restlessness, 38, 42, 56, 65 – 66
right dosage, 10 – 11
right remedies, 5, 9, 10, 43
Roemheld Syndrome, 84
sciatica, 66 – 67
shoulder pain, 67, 68
sleeplessness, 59 – 60, 86
sore throat, 75 – 76
stomachache, 12, 69 – 70
strains, sprains, 68 – 69
suffocation, feeling of, 35
sunburn, 71 – 72
sunstroke, 72 – 74
suppuration, 13 – 15, 29
travel sickness, 76
voice loss, 78
vomiting, 35, 49, 51, 52, 72, 79, 94
weather sensitivity, 80

About the Authors

Michael Helfferich is a pharmacist and naturopath in private practice in Markt Indersdorf, Germany. For many years now, his main emphasis has been on homeopathy. He holds seminars on this subject in Europe.

Walther Hohenester is a pharmacist and the author of numerous nonfiction books.

Important

Athough the information in this book has been very carefully researched and edited, neither the authors nor the publishers can accept responsibility for any detriment or harm resulting from the practical advice given herein.

Illustrations

Archiv für Kunst und Geschichte, Berlin: 6; Botanik-Bildarchiv Laux, Biberach: 13, 34, 37, 41, 49, 56, 53, 81, 83; Christian Weise Verlag, Munich: 14, 71; Das Fotoarchiv, Essen: 1; Hochleitner Rupert Dr., Munich: 93; Rehm, Claudia, Munich: 5